CCM NORTH TRAFFORD

The Art of Nails

The Art of Nails

A comprehensive style guide to nail treatments and nail art

Jacqui Jefford

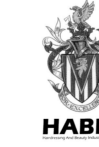

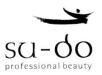

su-do
professional beauty

CREATIVE
NAIL DESIGN™

HABIA
Hairdressing And Beauty Industry Authority

THOMSON
™

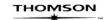

Austraila • Canada • Mexico • Singapore • Spain • United Kingdom • United States

THOMSON

The Art of Nails: A Comprehensive Style Guide to Nail Treatments and Nail Art

Copyright © 2005 Thomson Learning

The Thomson logo is a registered trademark used herein under licence.

For more information, contact Thomson Learning, High Holborn House, 50–51 Bedford Row, London WC1R 4LR or visit us on the World Wide Web at: http://www.thomsonlearning.co.uk

British Library Cataloguing-in-Publication Data
A catalogue record for this book is available from the British Library

ISBN-13: 978-1-84480-146-2
ISBN-10: 1-84480-146-2

First edition published 2005 by Thomson Learning

Designed and typeset by LewisHallam

Printed in Italy by Canale

Contents

Credits

A special 'thank you' to my partner Sue, without whose inspiration this book would not have happened. I would also like to say a special thanks to James Cumpsty, who has the patience of a saint, and to Alex Fox, for being so supportive of everything I do. And of course Samantha Sweet for always being there for me over the years. Thanks guys.

Photography
James Cumpsty
John Stone

Products
Creative Nail Design
Designer Nails
Sudo Professional Beauty
KISS UK
K-Sa-Ra

Nail Technicians
Michelle Hardy
Anne Swain
Samantha Biddle, for her candy nails
Kelly Swain
Gemma Jones
Body Art – Emilio

Hair
Essensuals Toni & Guy, Salisbury
Cor Kwakernaak

Make-up
Mandy Chauhan
Cor Kwakernaak
Karen Lockyer

Styling
Alex Fox of Scratch
Jane Bevan

Props
ASA Enterprises, Xiva Jewels, www.xivajewels.com, for gold nails
Repertoire Boutique, Salisbury
Confetti and Lace, Salisbury

Introduction

Working within the professional nail Industry over the last twenty years, I have seen the industry grow beyond belief. This is the first book of its kind within the industry. I hope that further books will be written on this subject so that this grows into a great reference library not only for nail professionals but also for other professionals with whom we work with such as make-up and hair artists, stylists, editors and photographers.

It was difficult deciding which styles should be included. After much deliberation it was easy to see that we should select those which give out the message that nail treatments are for everyone, male and female, young and old, serious and fun. I hope that message has been put across and that you enjoy the book.

Thank you

Jacqui

Foreword

At last the world of fashion and beauty can feast upon imagery that finishes the look. Yes, *finishes*, because no complete look is truly complete until the nails are groomed. This is the message the nail industry has been struggling to get heard for years as the make-up and hair industries have been riding their waves of style success and recognition.

This book has been a long time coming and is a true testament to the incredible work that the nail industry and its forward-thinking style leaders have been producing for many years.

It is with great pleasure that I introduce this fantastic nail style tome, which offers a delicious menu of nail designs for the avid nail technician as well as those who simply love the world of nail art and design.

As a close industry colleague and a friend I have worked alongside Jacqui Jefford for six years now, and in this time I have watched her industry profile flourish. Notwithstanding her sheer hard work, sweat and tears, Jacqui has emerged in the nail industry as a phoenix from the flames and stamped her mark across every sector imaginable, educating and pushing back the style boundaries. It is therefore appropriate that the first publication of this calibre should be produced by this industry icon.

Delivering nail design in a new and dynamic format, this is the most enlightening finger fashion fiesta you have ever seen: hold your breath, sit back and enjoy!

Alex Fox
Editor, *Scratch* magazine

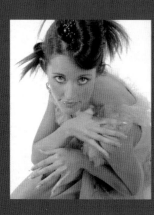
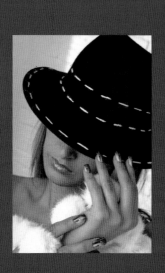
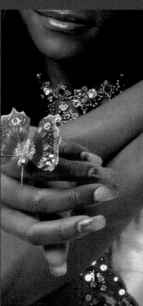
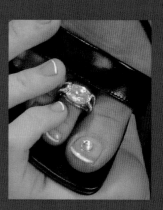

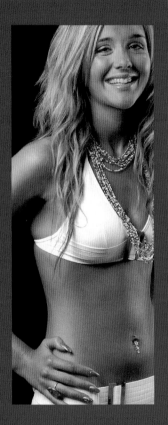

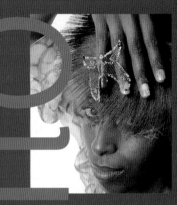

fashion

fashion

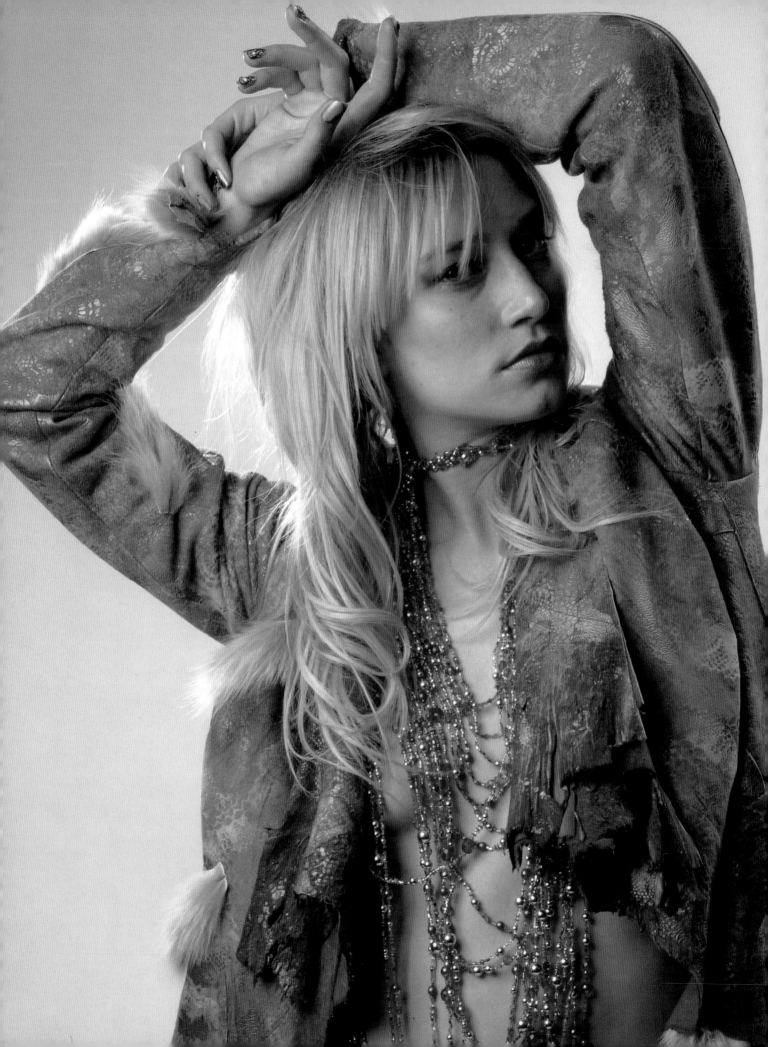

Fashion week

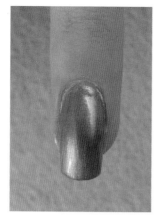 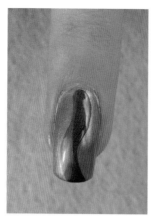 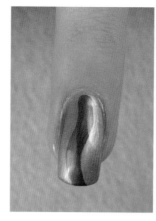 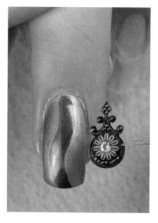

1 Base coat nails with Stickey base coat. Apply two coats of Creative Insomnia Enamel.

2 Using Creative Seduction Enamel paint a line down the centre of the nail using an enamel brush.

3 Using Creative Pharoah Gold Enamel apply to edge of nail beyond the middle colour. You may need to do another light coat to achieve colour depth.

4 Use a pair of tweezers to take the sticky-backed decal off the backing paper.

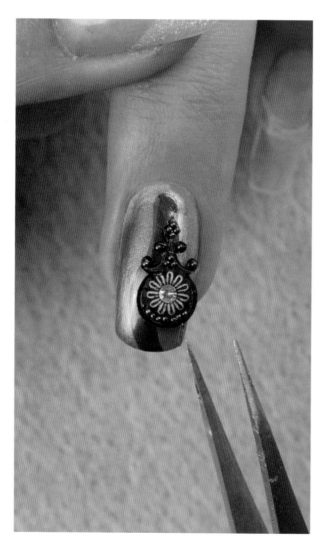

5 Place decal just off centre on the nail and press firmly into polish.

6 Be careful not to smudge the polish when positioning the decal. This look is quick and easy to do when you are at a venue such as London Fashion Week and you need to do a design really quickly. The decal could also be embedded in acrylic for a great salon treatment.

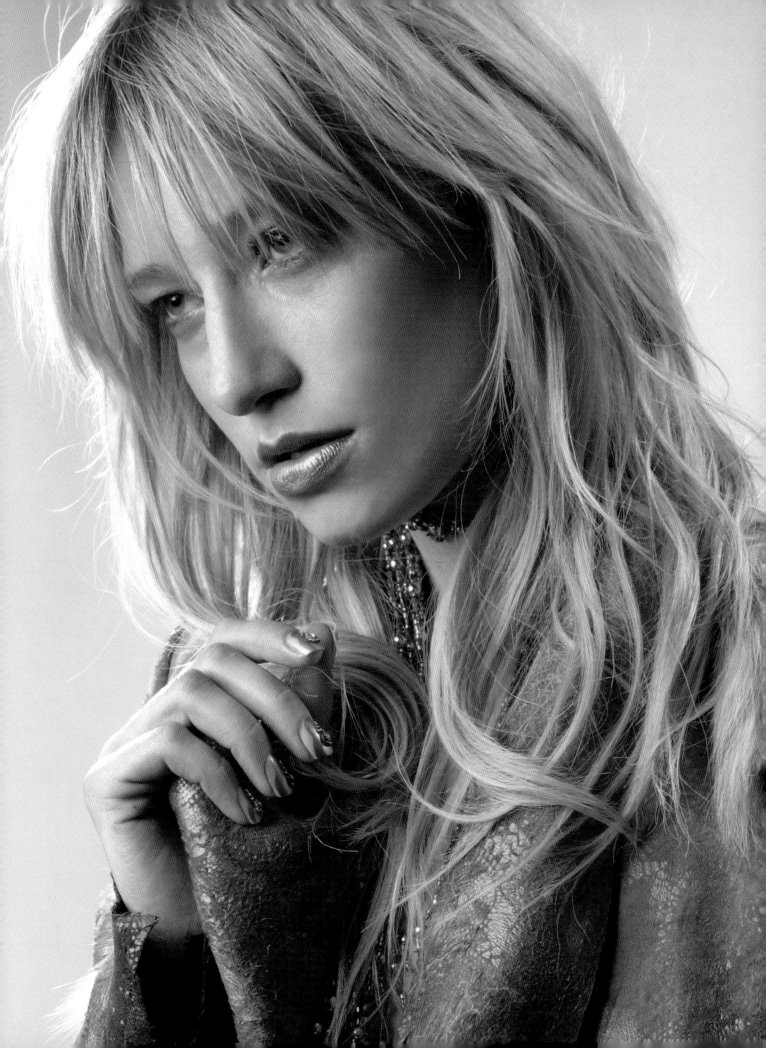

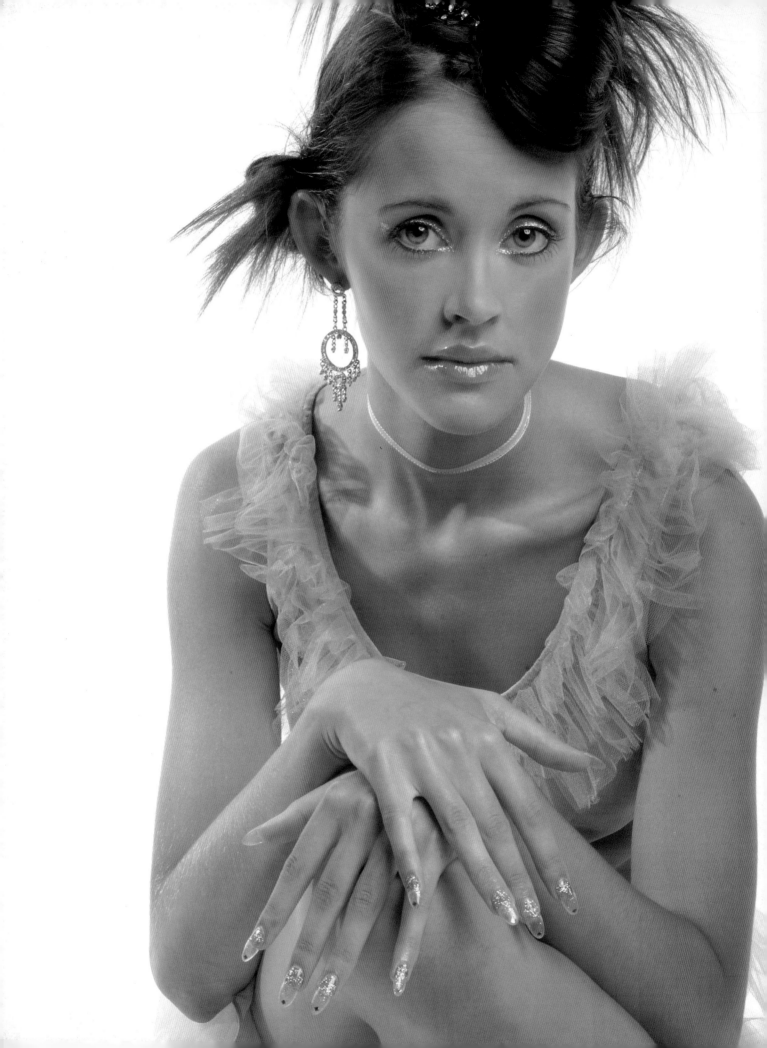

Party girl

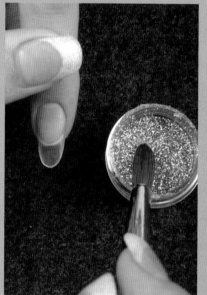

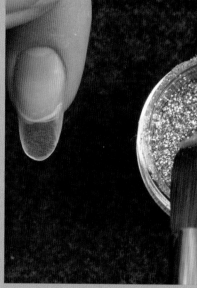

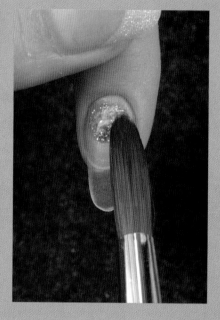

1 Apply, cut and blend a
Creative Clear Tip.

2 Take a bead of Creative
Perfect Clear Powder and scoop
it into pale green glitter.

3 Apply to cuticle end of nail
and pull bead down the nail.

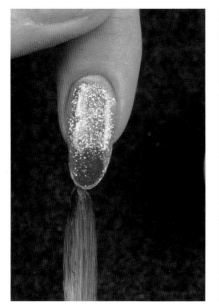

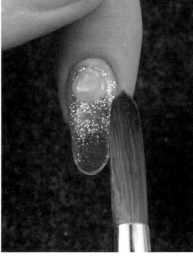

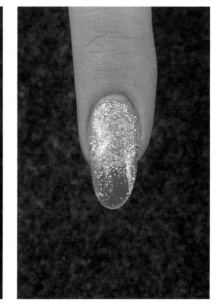

4 Pulling the bead down the nail gives a lovely fade: thick glitter ending in fine glitter particles on the free edge.

5 Apply a thin bead of Creative Perfect Clear and cover entire nail.

6 Ensure the nail is completely covered with product before buffing. Buff the nails to a high shine using appropriate files and finishing with Girlfriend Buffer.

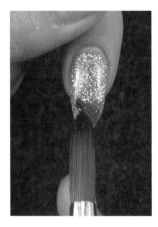 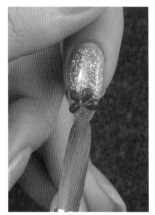 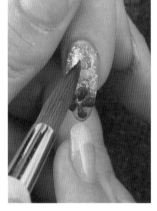

7 Custom blend the Mosaic Powders, using three parts Spanish tile and one part Black, to create a deep red colour powder. Apply a small bead to the lower part of the nail and pull into a petal shape.

8 Repeat until red petals are complete.

9 Taking small beads of Creative Golden Glass Mosaic Powder create small beads moving upwards towards the cuticle. Beads should get smaller as they reach the top.

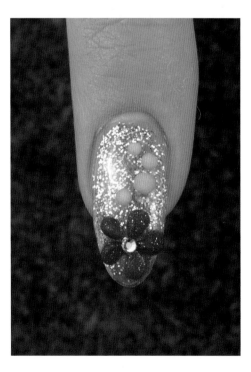

10 Use either another colour bead for the final centre of the flower or a rhinestone in a complementary colour.

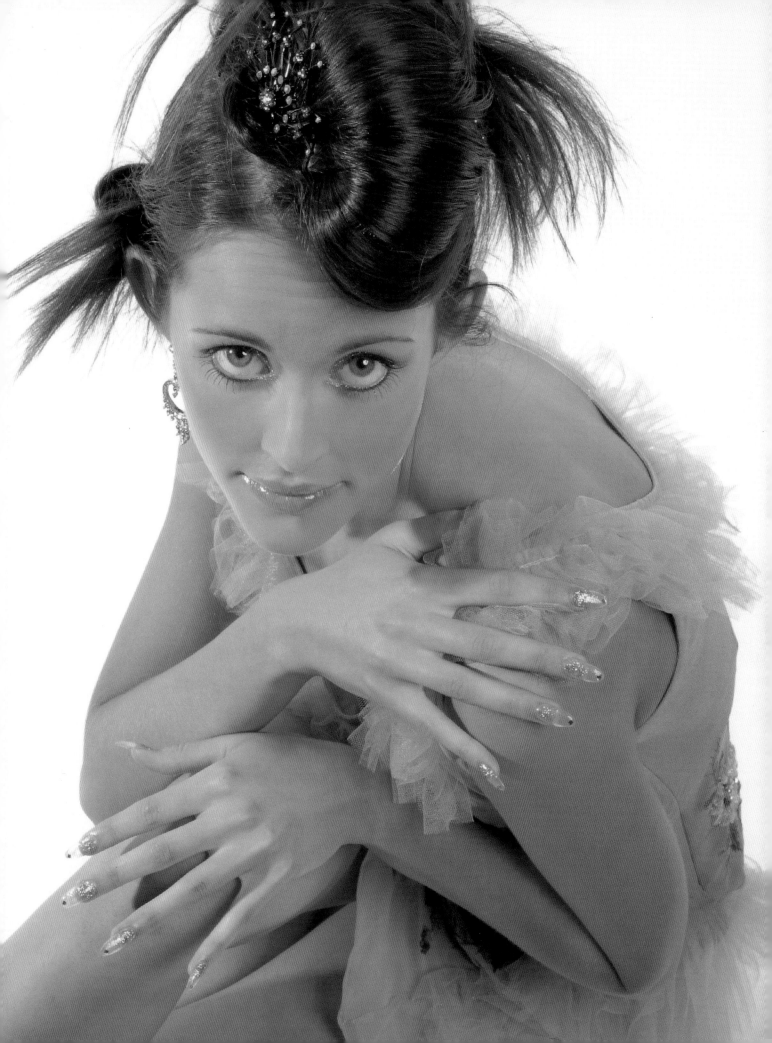

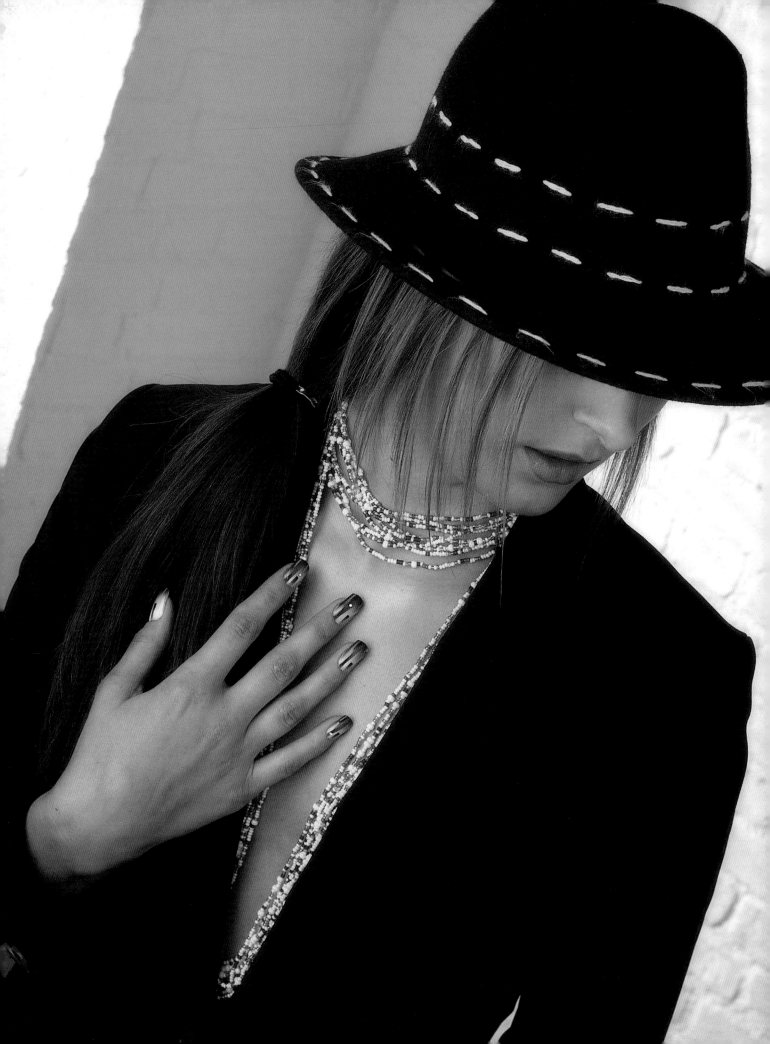

Rock chick

Rock chick

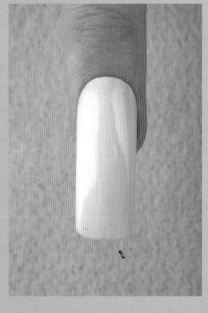

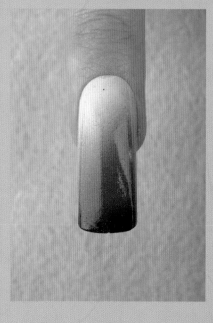

1 Apply base coat to nails. Using an airbrush spray Sudo opaque cream paint onto all nails.

2 Using Sudo opaque gold colour paint spray the free edge of the nail to three quarters of the way up, creating a colour fade.

3 Spray Sudo golden brown onto the edge of the nail to complete the colour fade.

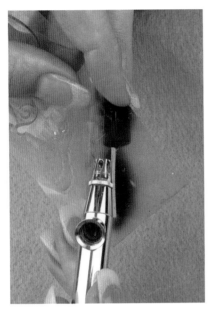 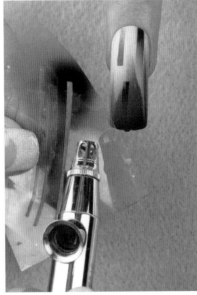 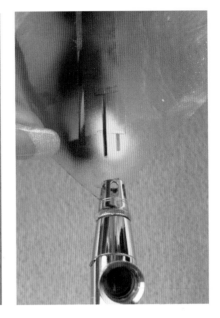

4 Hold a stencil on the cream top part of the nail and spray lightly through it with the Sudo darker brown colour.

5 Repeat again at the top and once at the bottom of the nail. When spraying, fade the line from dark to light to give the illusion of 3D.

6 Holding the same stencil but this time on the dark brown at the bottom, spray two small Sudo opaque cream paint lines.

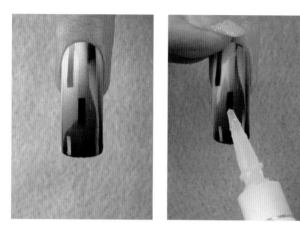

7 When spraying through stencils you must spray lightly otherwise the paint will leak under the stencil and spoil the design. At this stage seal the design with Sudo sealant and then top coat.

8 Apply a very small bead of Gel Bond adhesive to the middle of the darker lower line.

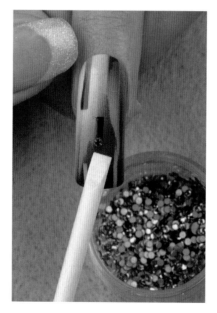

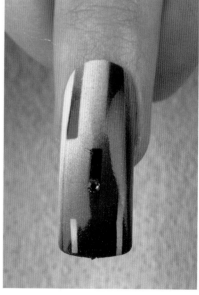

9 Using a dampened orange stick apply a small rhinestone to the Gel Bond.

10 Airbrush designs can be really versatile because of the technique of shading and blending. This design can be done with many different colour combinations to match clothes, accessories or even jewellery.

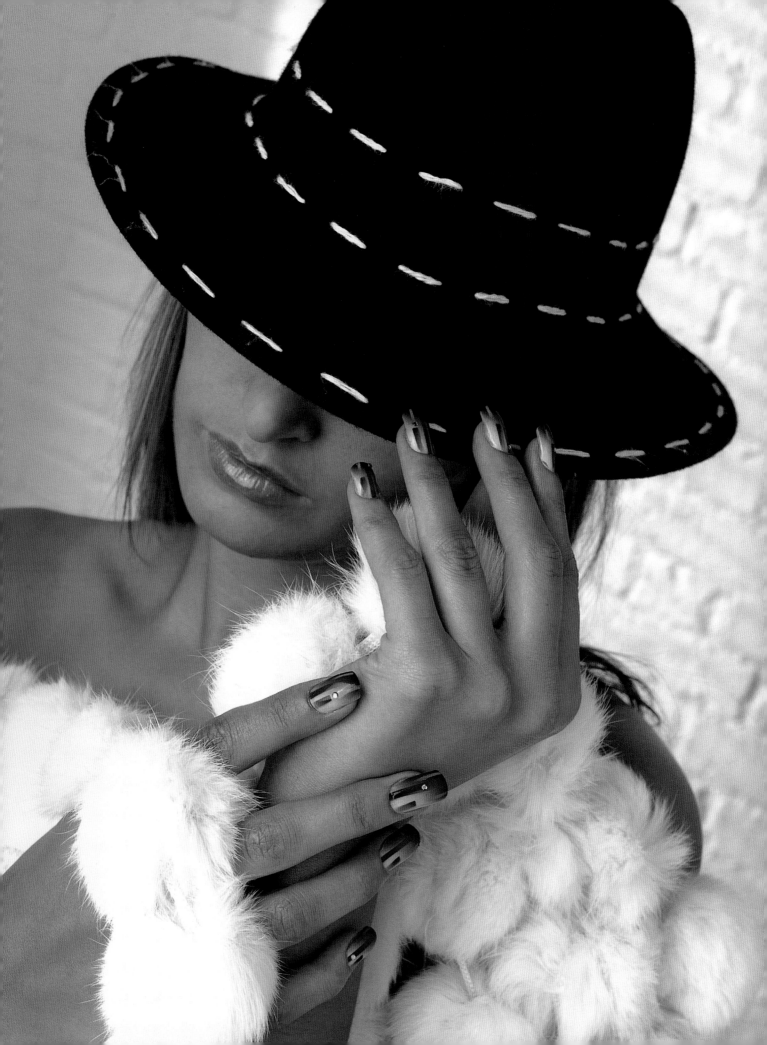

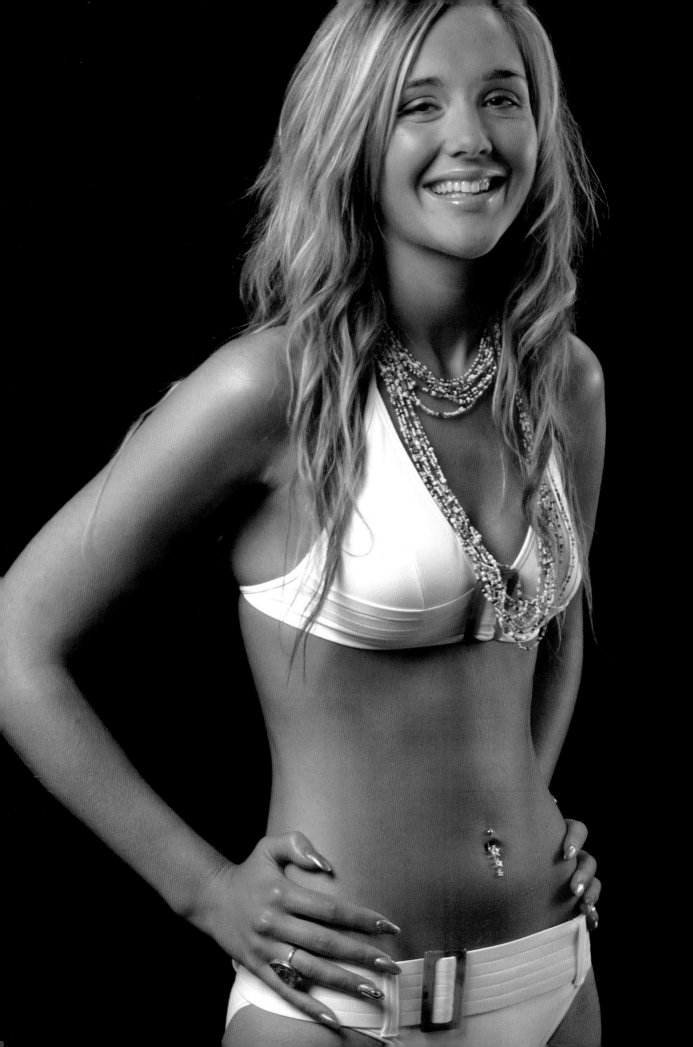

Beach babe

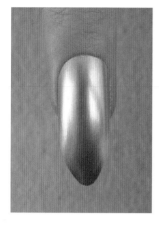

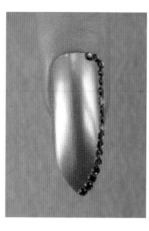

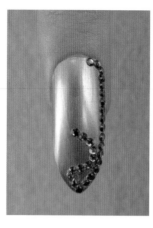

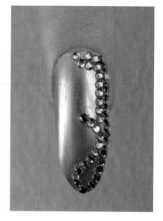

1 Base coat the nails with Sticky. Apply two coats of Creative Iced Cappucino Enamel.

2 Apply small dots of Gel Bond adhesive up the side of the nail from the free edge to the cuticle area. Apply amber rhinestones to the Gel Bond with a dampened orange stick.

3 Apply Gel Bond again, curling up from the free edge, and embed rhinestones onto the Gel Bond.

4 Start another line of rhinestones alongside the previous but make them a slightly different colour.

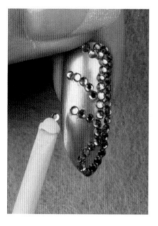

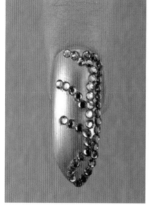

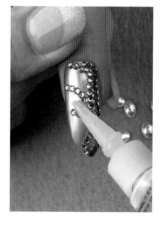

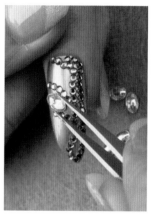

5 Adhere rhinestones in two lines coming out from the side. Leave enough space for cabouchons crystals.

6 Attach enough rhinestones to cover practically one half of the nail and choose rhinestone colours that complement the polish colour underneath.

7 Apply two beads of Gel Bond in between lines of rhinestones.

8 With tweezers place two large Swarvoski cabouchon crystals onto nail and hold until dry.

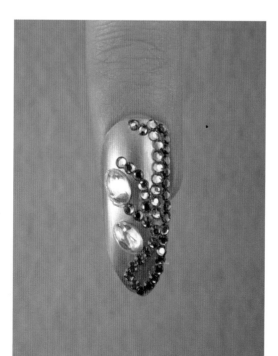

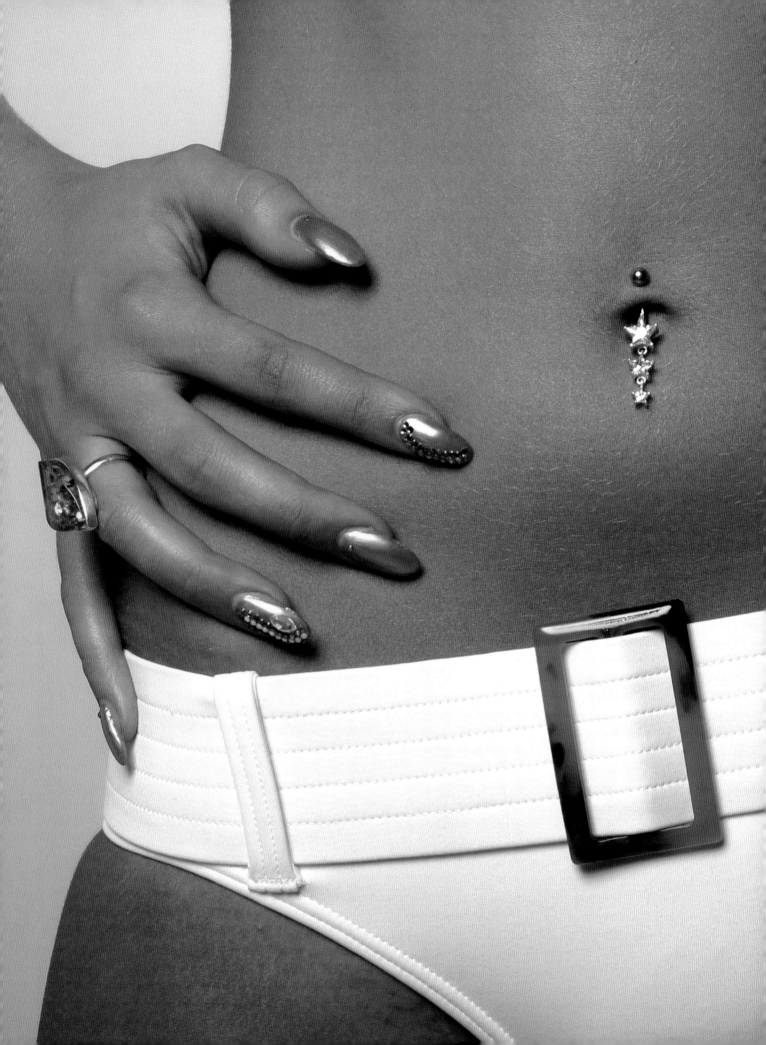

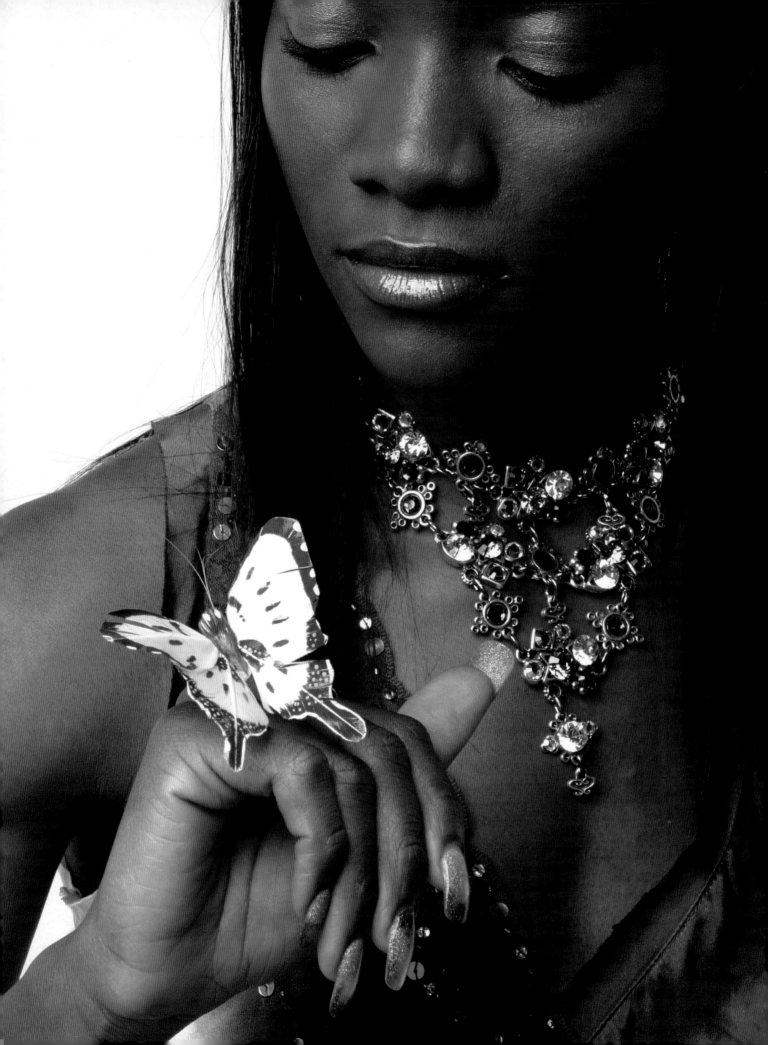

Garden party

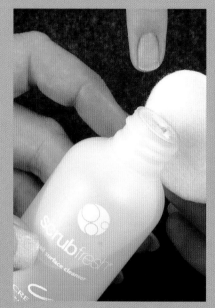

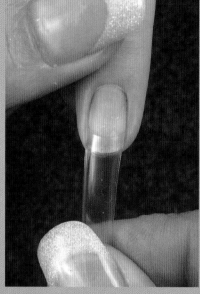

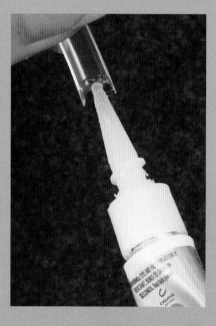

1 Prepare the natural nail for a tip. Perform cuticle work. Use Scrubfresh to dehydrate and cleanse the natural nail.

2 Take a Creative Clear Tip and size it to the natural nail.

3 Apply Gel Bond adhesive to the well in the tip and a little to the free edge of the nail.

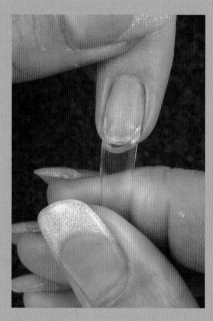

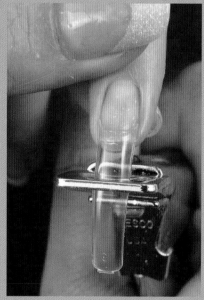

4 Apply tip to free edge of nails ensuring pressure is enough for adhesive to bond properly to natural nail.

5 Cut and shape tip to required length and desired shape.

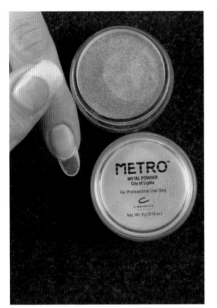

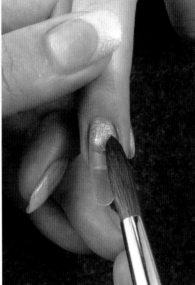

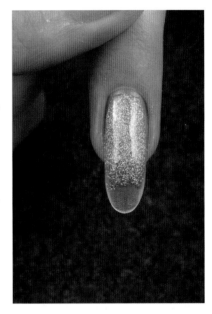

6 Blend tip to natural nail carefully and gently so that it cannot be detected.

7 Using Creative City of Lights Metro Powder and Retention + create a bead and apply it to the cuticle area of nail, blending down to the middle.

8 Ensure that the blend fades into nothing two thirds down the nail. This will help the colour blend.

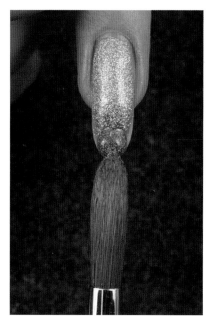 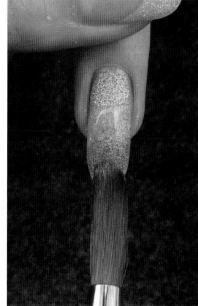 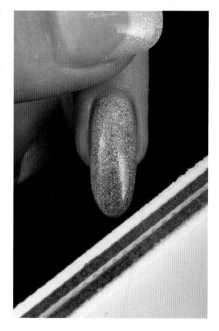

9 Take a small bead of Creative The Golden City Metro Powder and apply it to the free edge of the nail pushing bead gently up towards the silver. Leave the bulk of the gold at the free edge and blend the two colours.

10 Apply a small layer of Creative Perfect Clear Powder over entire nail.

11 Buff the nails up to a high shine finishing with the Girlfriend Buffer and Solar Oil.

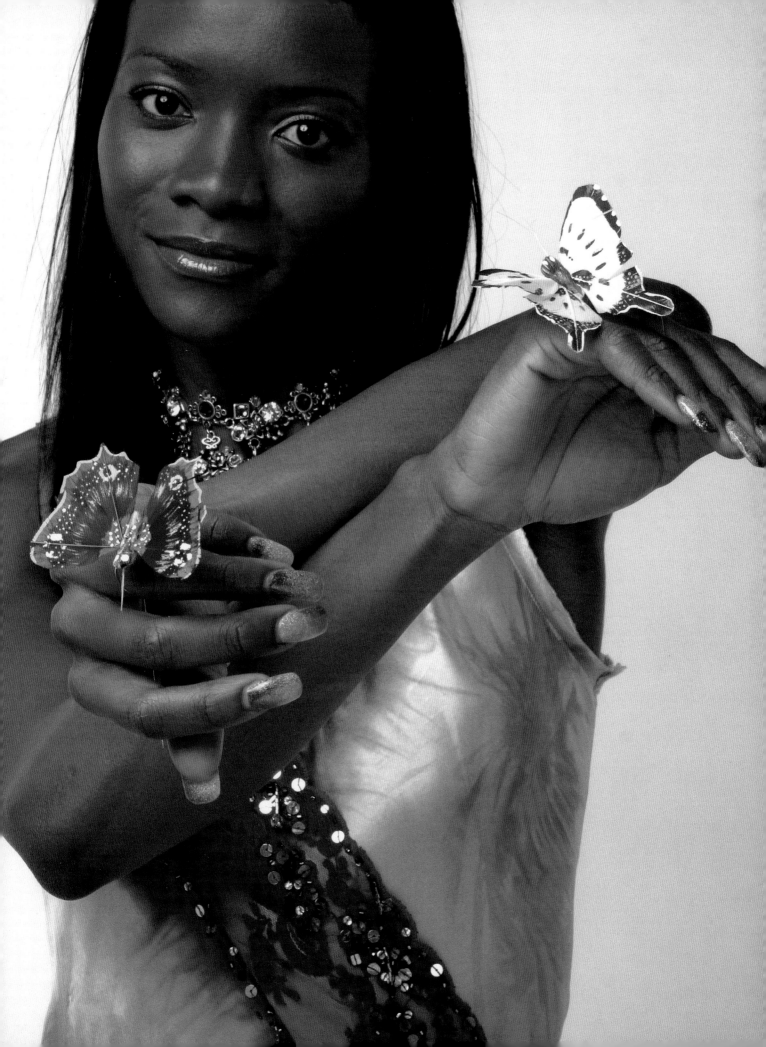

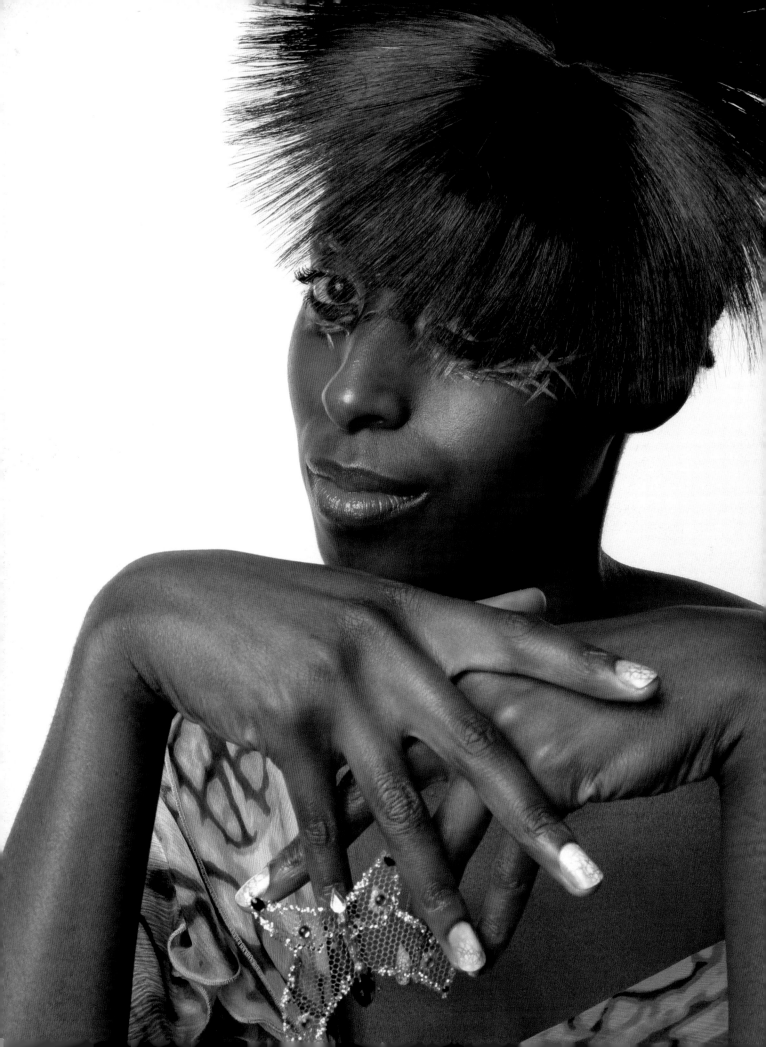

Dragonfly

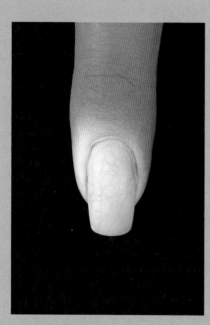

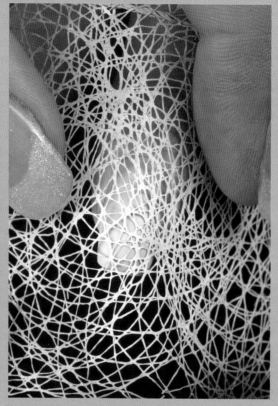

1 Airbrush nine nails with Sudo light blue opaque paint. Hold a stencil over the top and spray through it with a slightly darker colour.

2 Top coat all nine nails and clean off the paint around the cuticle.

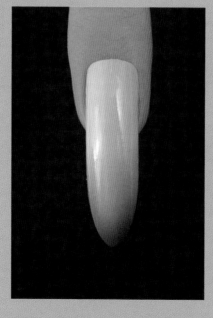

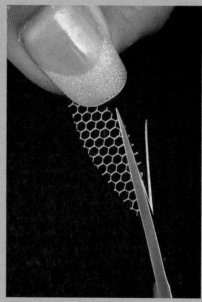

3 Airbrush the tenth nail with Sudo light blue to dark blue colour fade.

4 Using a blue net cut out four dragonfly wings.

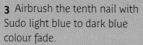

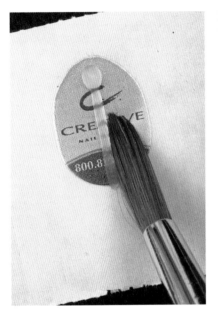

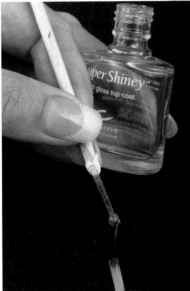

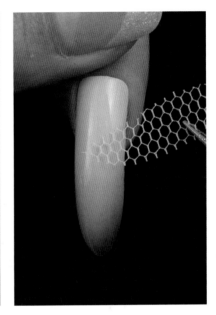

5 On a sculpting form create the body of a dragonfly with Creative Perfect Clear Powder.

6 Coat dragonfly body with Super Shiney top coat and dip it into a glitter pot to cover with dark blue glitter.

7 Apply a small bead of Gel Bond to the centre of the nail and apply all four wings to the Gel Bond. Hold in place and use an activator spray to set the Gel Bond.

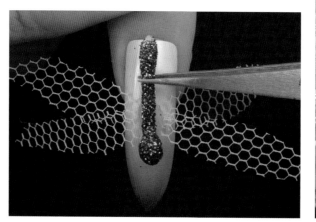

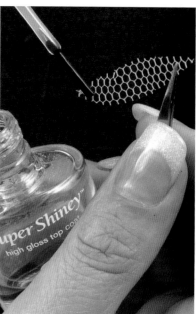

8 Apply a couple of small beads of acrylic along where the body will set and hold it in place until it is set.

9 Apply Super Shiney to the wing tips and dip them into the glitter pot. This can be done before the wings are applied to the nail or after.

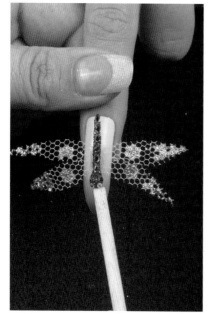

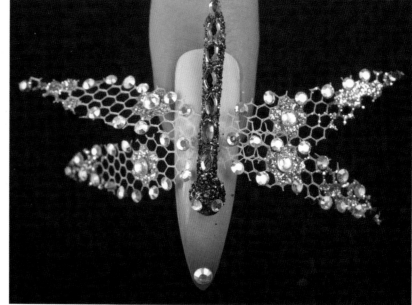

10 Apply small amounts of Gel Bond along the back of dragonfly and for its eyes place variously coloured rhinestones in place using a dampened orange stick.

11 Add more rhinestones to the wings using small amounts of Super Shiney. You will see from the main picture that you can create butterflies or any other creatures with a little imagination.

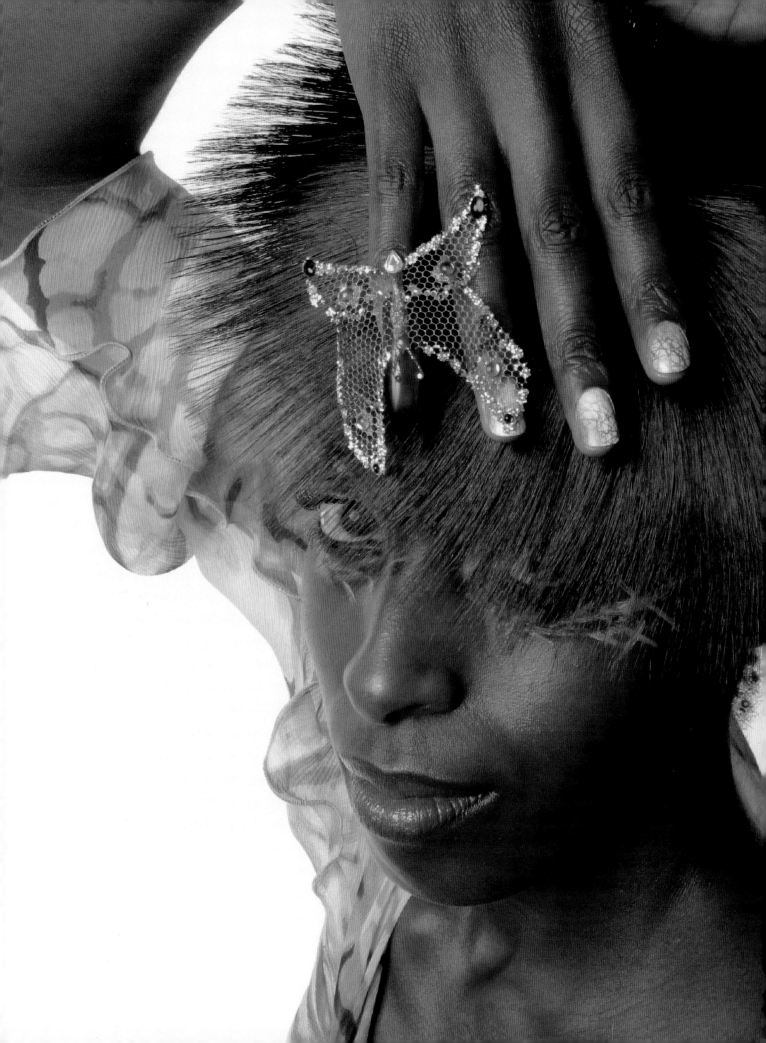

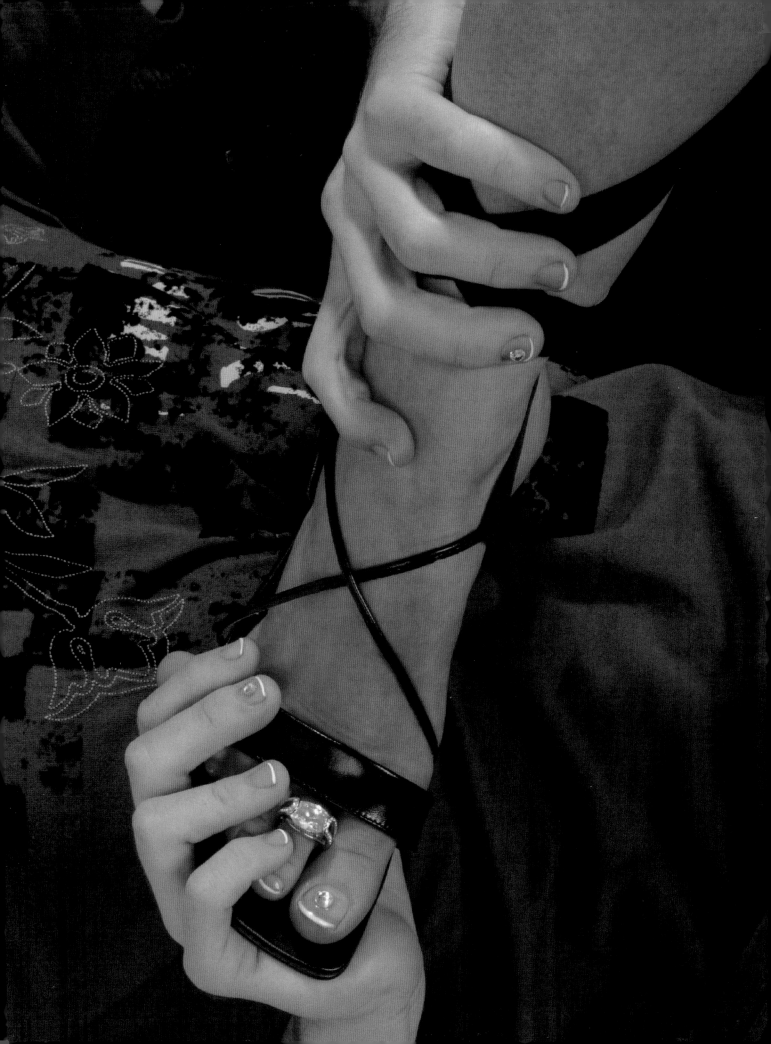

His & hers bling

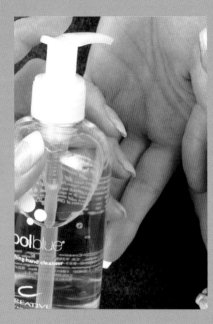

1 Use Cool Blue to sanitise you and your client's hands.

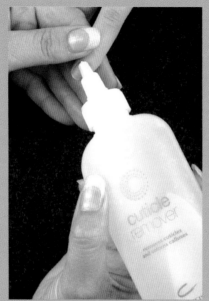

2 Apply Creative Cuticle Remover, push back cuticle and remove any excess. Wash off cuticle remover and dry the client's hands.

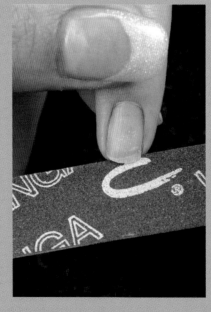

3 File nails to shape and length required.

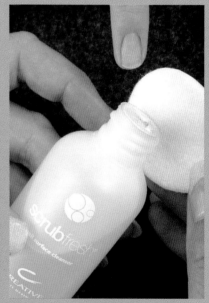

4 Using Scrubfresh and a pad remove all oil from the nail plate.

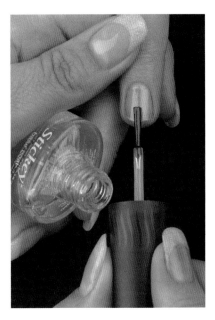 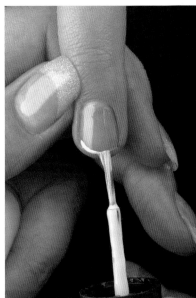 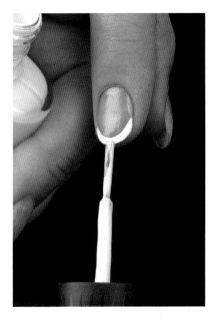

5 Apply a coat of Stickey base coat.

6 Using Creative Cream Puff Enamel, apply a thin coat along free edge of nail.

7 Go back again and take line slightly higher. Make sure the French line is curved and not straight across.

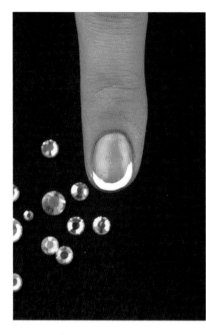 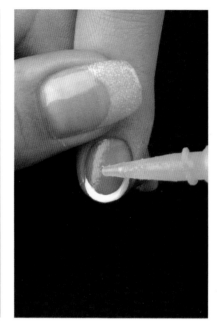 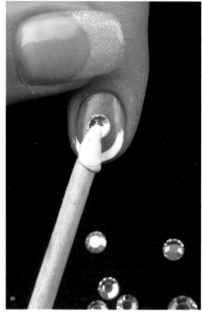

8 Neaten up the line if necessary with a fine art brush and some Scrubfresh and then top coat with Super Shiney.

9 Apply a small amount of Gel Bond Adhesive to the middle of the finger and toenail.

10 Using a orange stick tipped with blue tac position a large rhinestone onto Gel Bond.

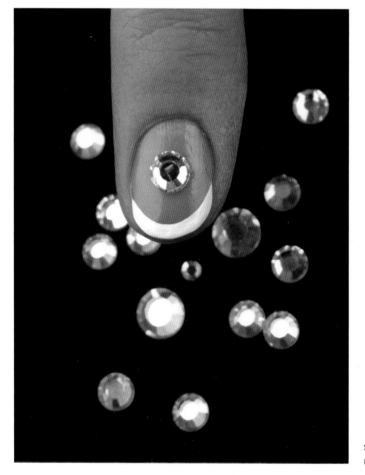

11 Hold rhinestone in place until dry.

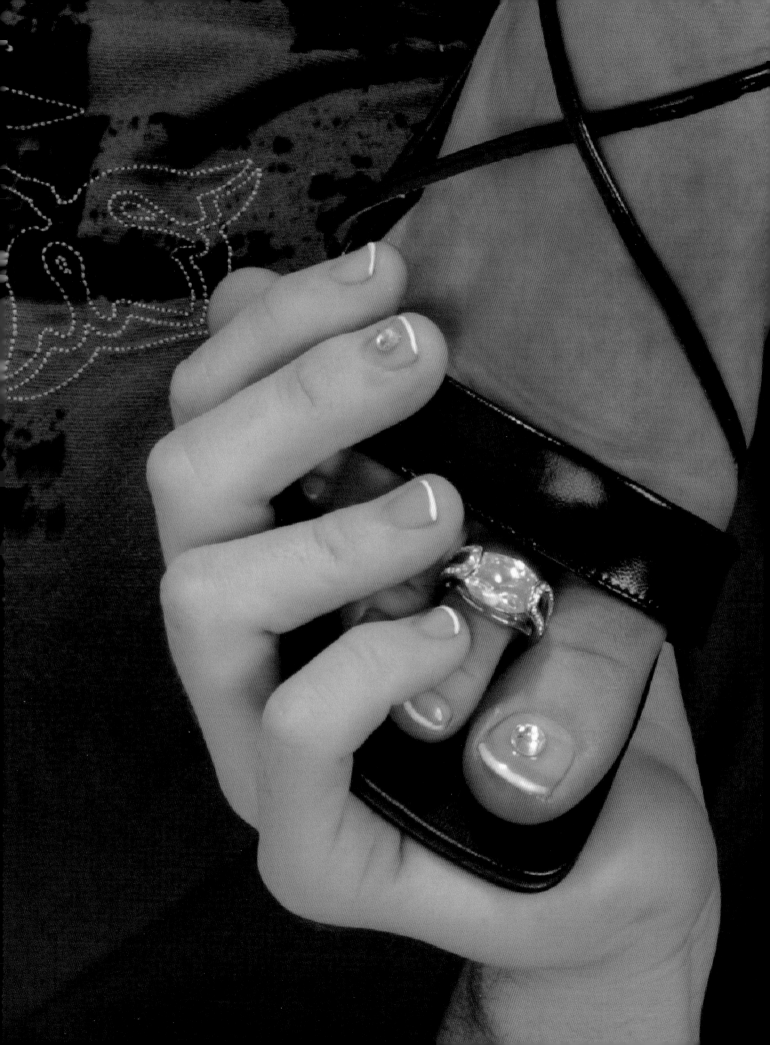

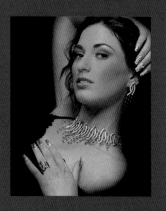
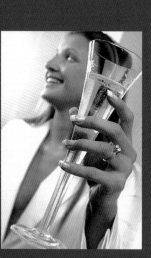
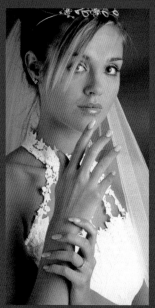

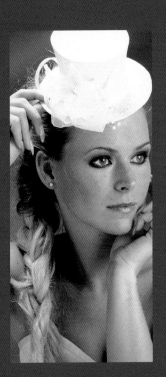

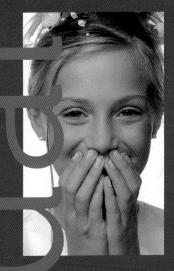

bridal

- Hen night
- Wedding guest
- Traditional bride
- Alternative bride
- Asian bride
- Bridesmaid

bridal

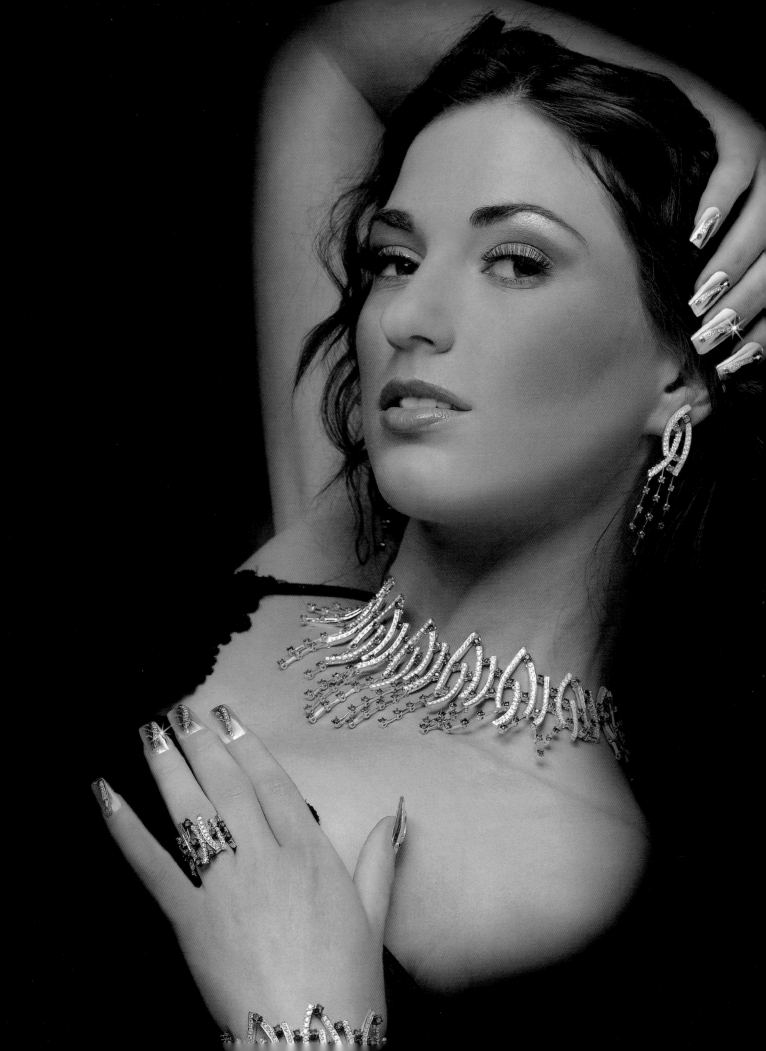

Hen night

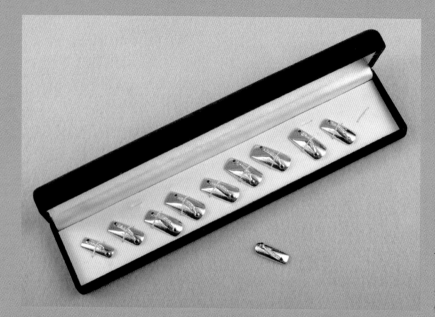

1 These are solid white gold nails with diamonds and sapphires. They can be worn just for the night or more permanently for a week or two. If longer wear is required they should be applied by a qualified technician.

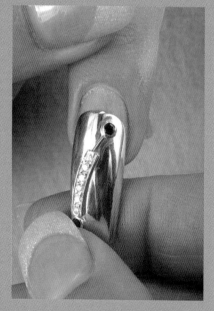

2 Either one nail or a whole set can be applied depending on the look you want. Ensure that you size each gold nail to the size of the natural nail. Go slightly larger rather than smaller if the size is inbetween.

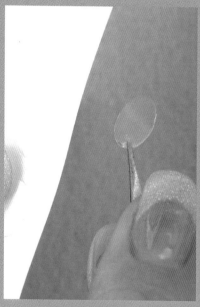

3 Take a nail bandage, which is a small piece of sticky-backed clear plastic.

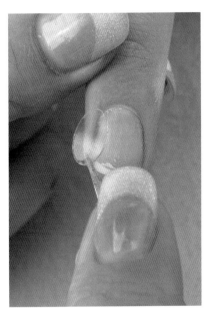 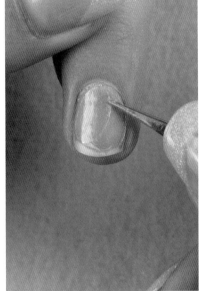 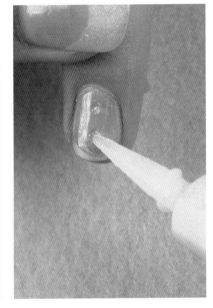

4 Size the bandage to ensure it fits nail. Two or three may have to be used on larger nails. Peel off backing paper with tweezers.

5 Apply to clean, oil-free nail plate with tweezers and press down with finger. If you hold the bandage with your fingers you will lose the sticky base on the back and it will not adhere properly to the nail plate.

6 Apply two to three dots of Gel Bond adhesive to the bandage coated nail plate. Larger nails may need double the amount.

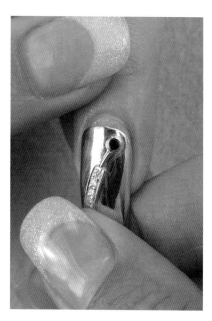

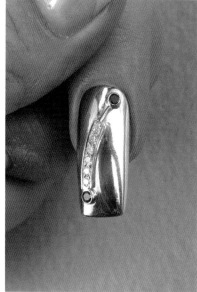

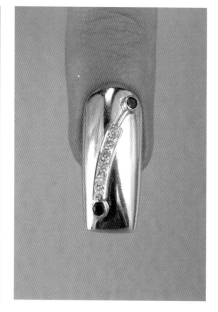

7 Take a gold nail and press firmly into place on nail plate. Try not to move once the nail is in place as the adhesive has started to set and you will disturb the process.

8 Wait for ten seconds and ensure the nail is set. If you want a more permanent application you can adhere the nail straight onto the nail plate with Gel Bond, but it must then be removed with product remover or acetone.

9 When buying nails of this quality ensure they are a good fit and that when they are applied it is done properly otherwise it could be a costly purchase. There are many colours, precious stones and designs to choose from and as you will see from the picture you can have nails to match your jewellery.

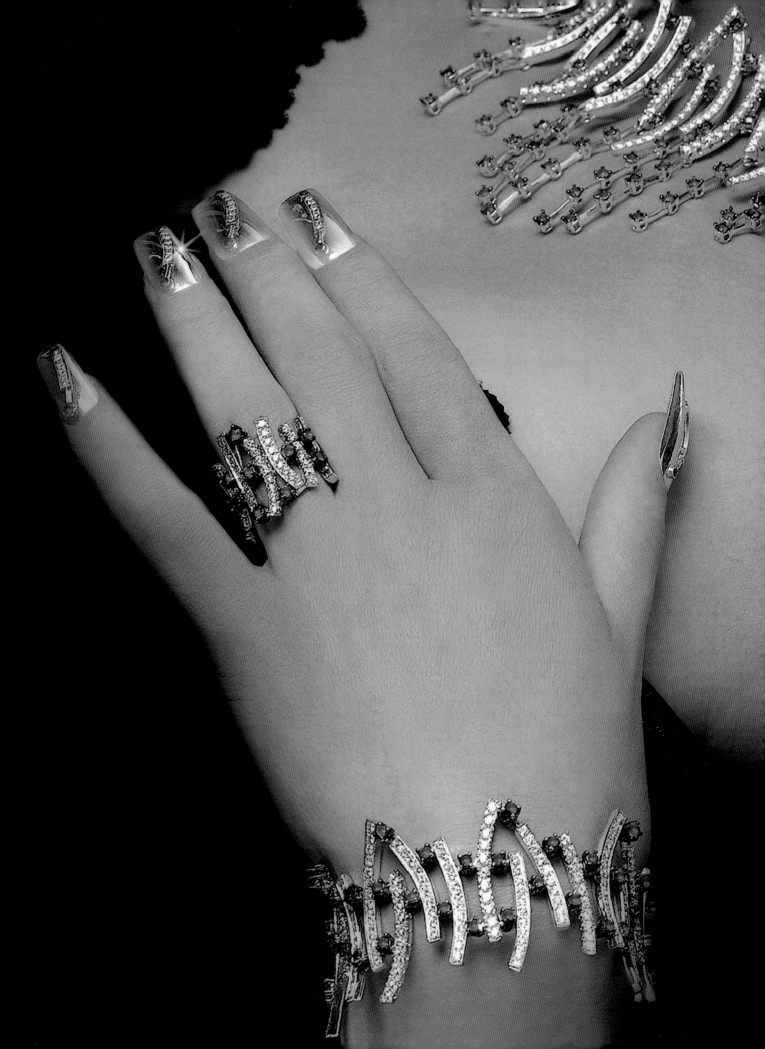

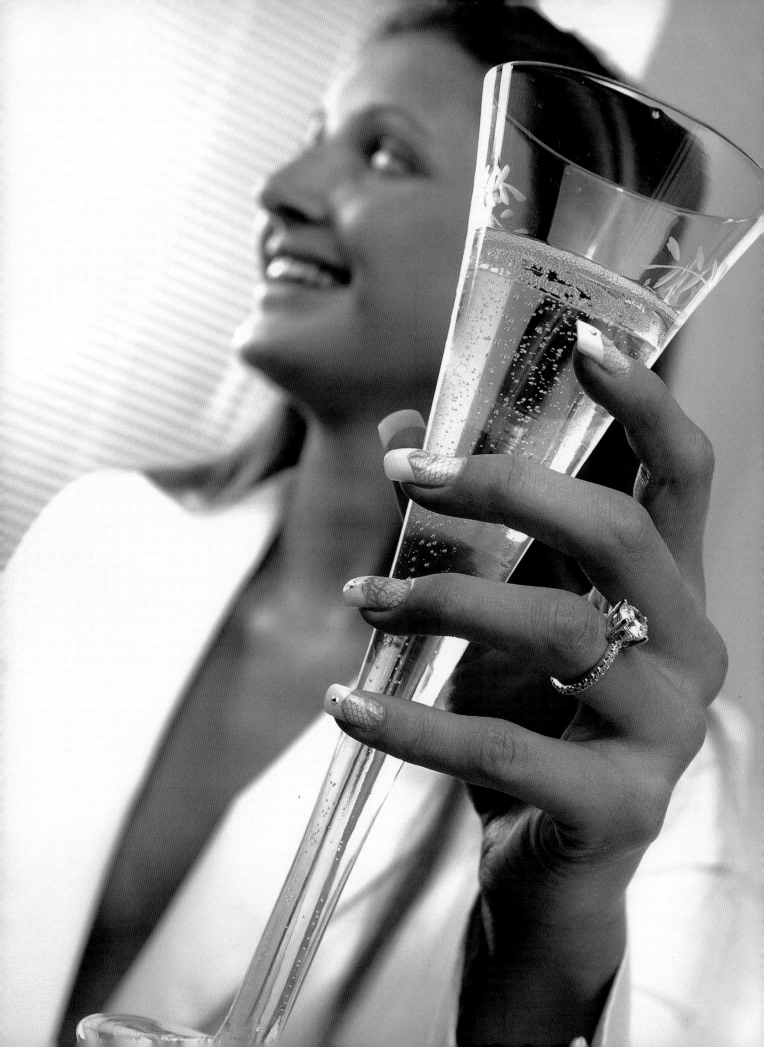

Wedding guest

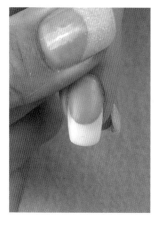 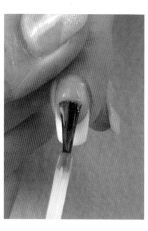 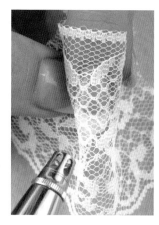 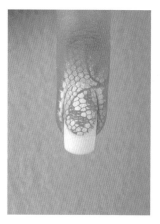

1 This design is one of the quickest to do and looks stunning on a French polish.

2 Use a good base coat. This design uses an airbrush although it could be done carefully with a white paint. It would take much longer for a hand painted nail to dry.

3 Find a fine piece of lace and practise first before you work on a client. Once ready hold the lace over the nail plate firmly and spray lightly, building up Sudo white paint through the lace.

4 Remove lace carefully. If you do not like the look it is easy to remove paint and spray again within a minute.

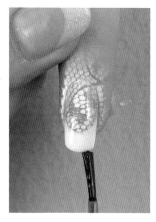 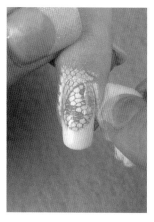 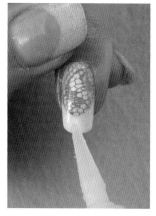 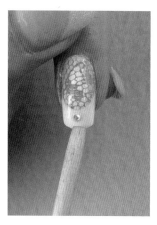

5 Apply sealant for the airbrush paint you are using. Wait for it to dry and then apply a top coat.

6 Remove paint from skin with Scrubfresh or non-acetone polish remover. Try not to go too close to the nail. Any excess will wash off of the skin when nails are dry.

7 If you want to add some decoration apply a small bead of Gel Bond Adhesive to the middle of the white edge.

8 Using a damp orange stick pick up a rhinestone and place onto small bead of Gel Bond Adhesive, pressing into place.

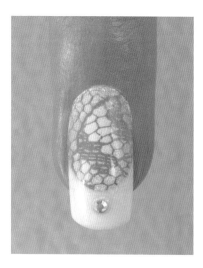

9 This design also looks good if you use red or black paint for a honeymoon break.

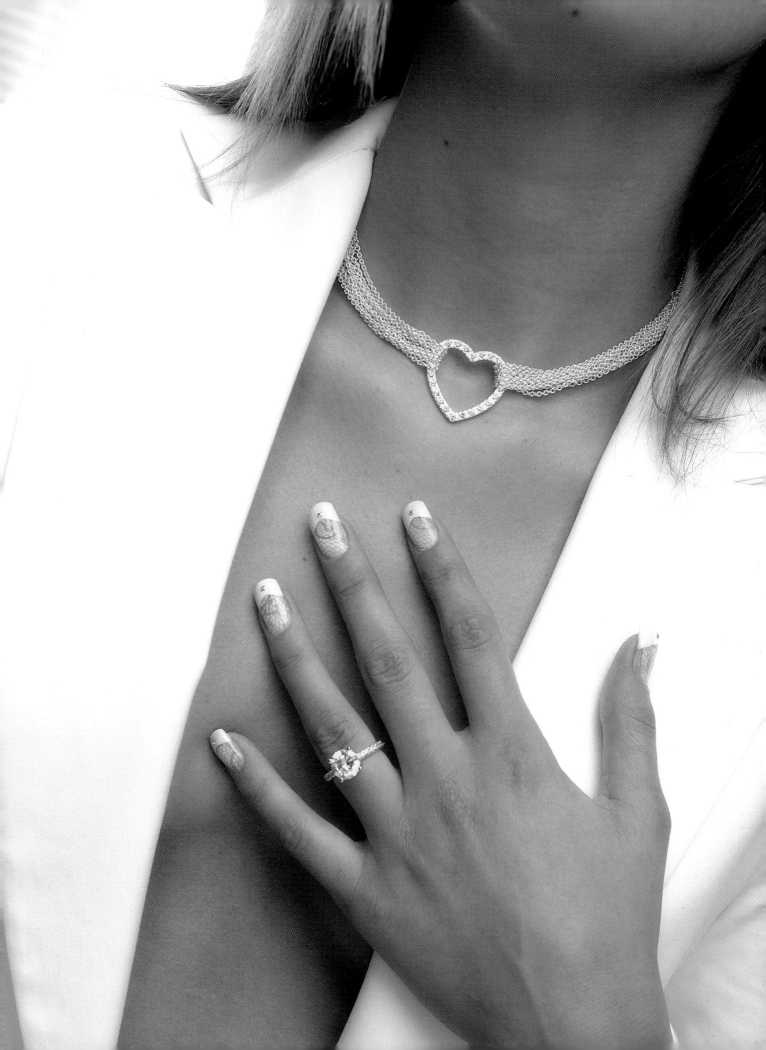

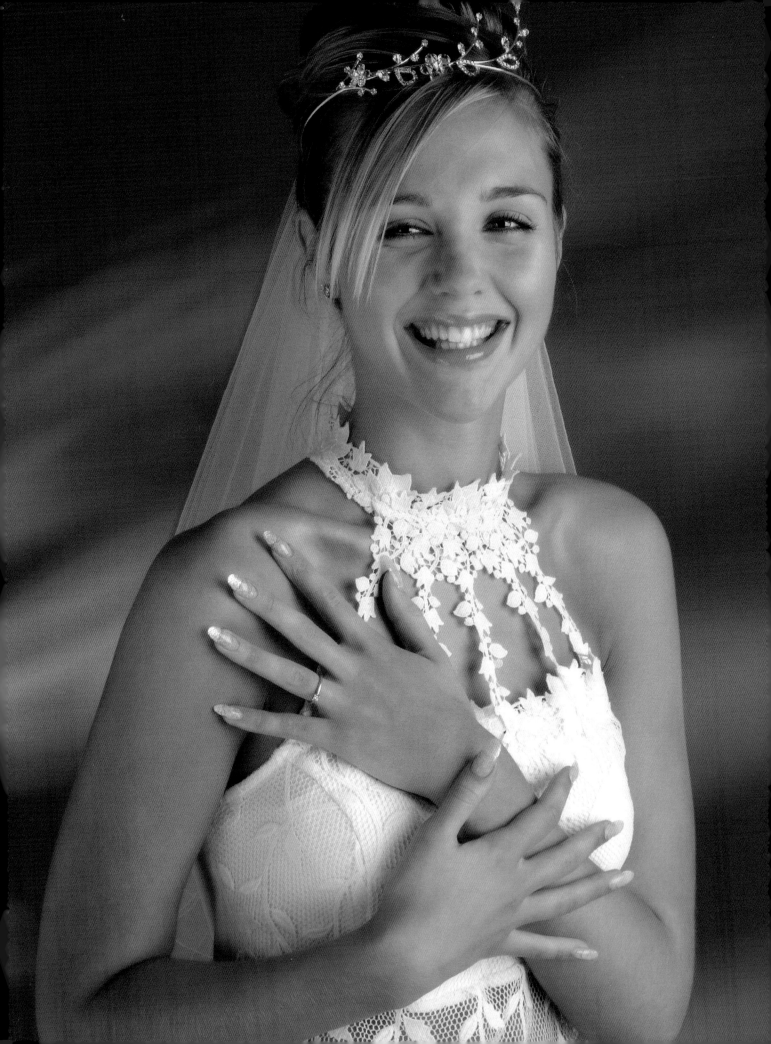

Traditional bride

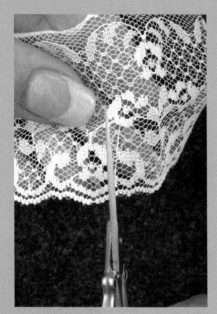

1 This design is using lace embedded within acrylic nails and is a more permanent bridal look. It looks more effective if used on clear tips.

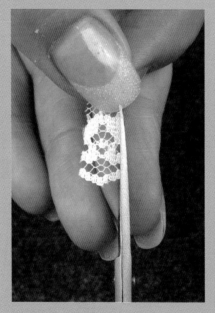

2 Take a piece of lace and cut it to shape matching the whole nail plate.

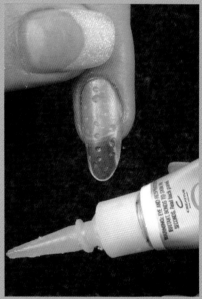

3 Ensure nail plate is cleansed using Scrubfresh and apply a few small dots of Gel Bond Adhesive.

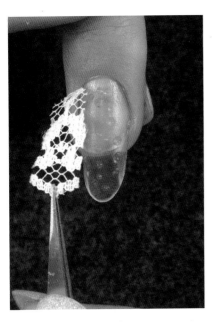

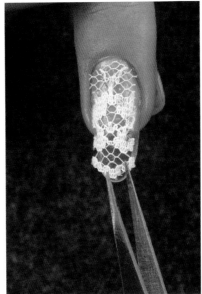

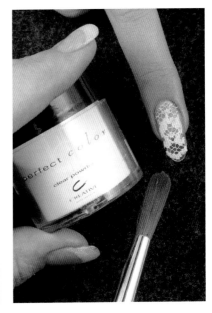

4 With tweezers apply lace onto nail plate.

5 Press down with tweezers, ensuring all edges are in contact with Gel Bond.

6 Using Perfect Clear Powder and Retention + apply acrylic over lace.

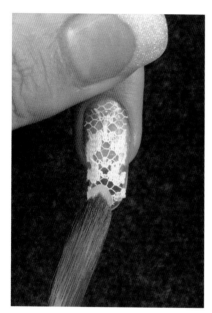 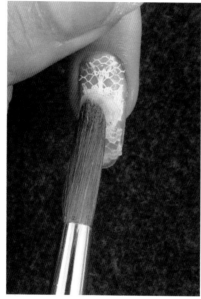 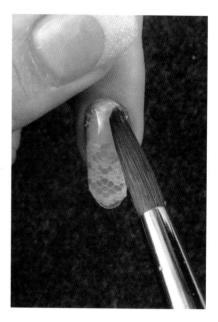

7 Starting off at the free edge make sure that the bead of acrylic penetrates the lace to ensure a good bond to the nail plate.

8 Ensure the acrylic covers the whole nail without going onto the surrounding soft tissue. This can easily be achieved by working the beads into the three nail zones, free edge, apex and cuticle area.

9 Once product has been applied to the whole the nail, you can buff down with appropriate files.

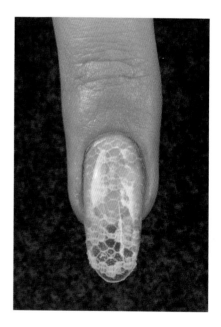

10 Bring all nails to a high shine using Girlfriend Buffer and finish with Solar Oil.

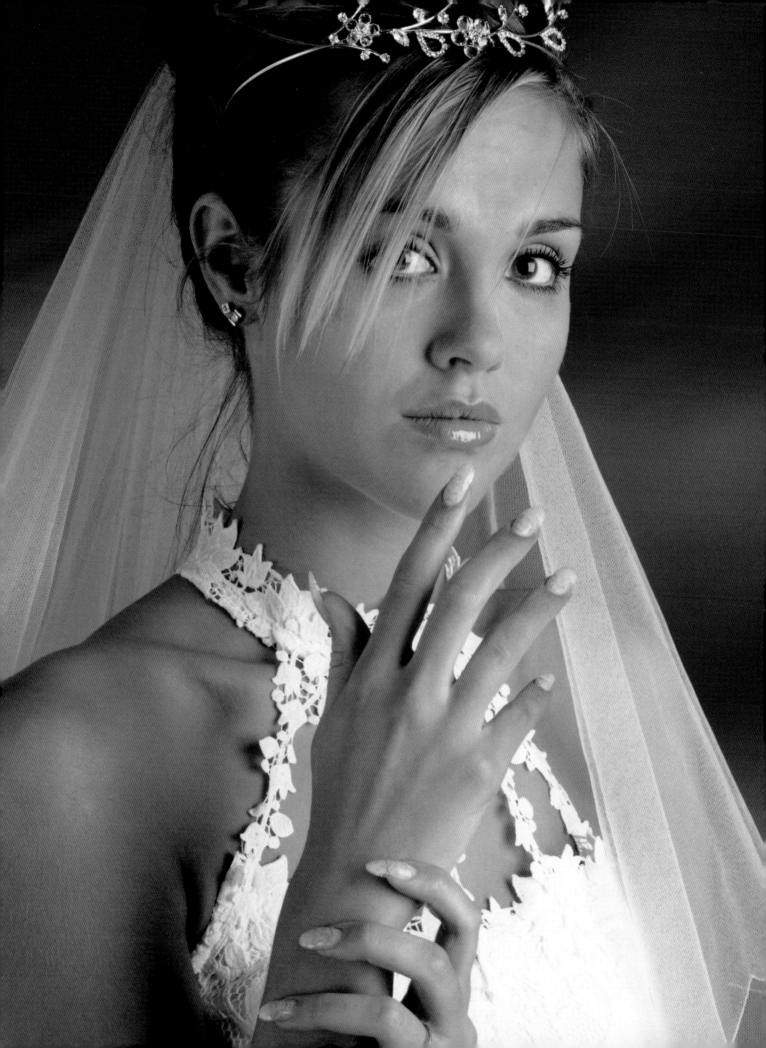

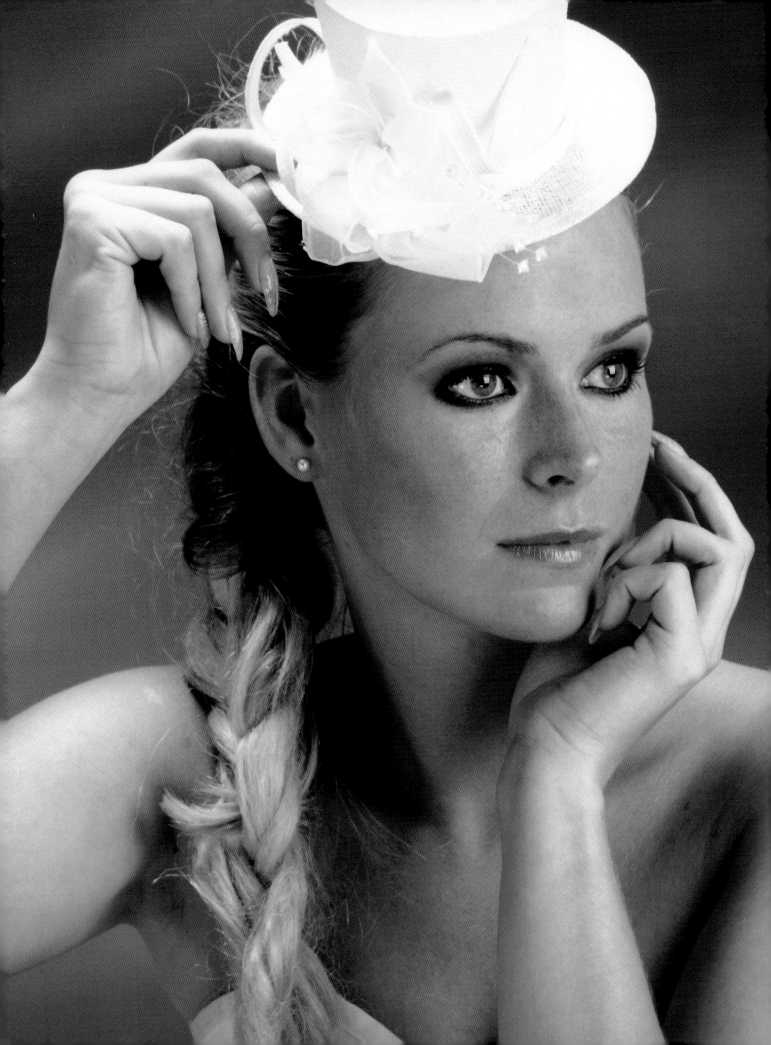

Alternative bride

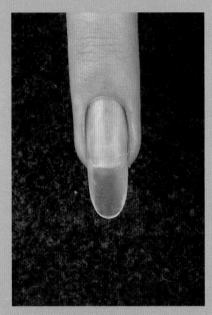

1 Apply a Creative Clear Tip,
blend to natuiral nail and
shape.

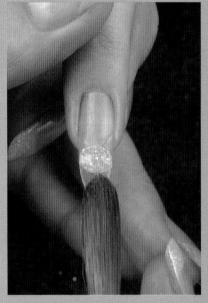

2 Use Scrubfresh to ensure
the nail is clean and dehydrated.
Apply a bead of Creative
Glimmer Powder with
Retention + to the free edge.

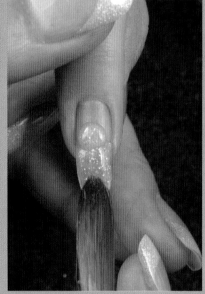

3 Work with the acrylic in all
three nail zones to achieve a
well-balanced nail.

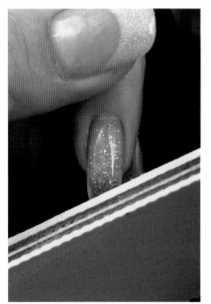

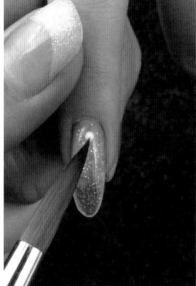

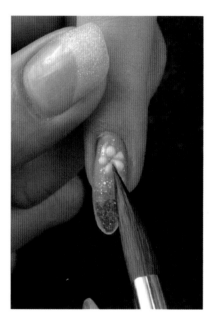

4 Buff nails into shape using appropriate files. Finish nails to a high shine using Creative Girlfriend Buffer.

5 Using Creative Perfect White Powder apply a very small dry bead to the corner of the nail.

6 Apply another four beads to form a flower. Ensure that the beads are dry and small. Allow them to settle and push them back into shape if you have to with your brush.

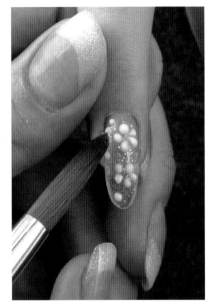

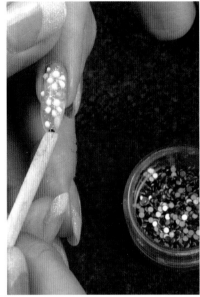

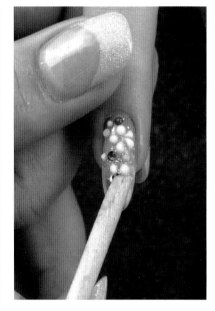

7 Apply two or three very small beads of Creative Mosaic Jade Powder to create leaves amongst the flowers.

8 The centre of the flowers can either be dots of Creative Mosaic Spanish Tile Powder or red rhinestones depending on what the bride wants.

9 Apply small beads of Gel Bond Adhesive onto the places where you want to position the rhinestones. Apply rhinestones with a dampened orange stick and press down into Gel Bond.

10 This design can be achieved with a variety of colours and looks. Lilies look great as well as daisies. Practise on tips first: this also gives you a portfolio of different looks from which your clients can choose.

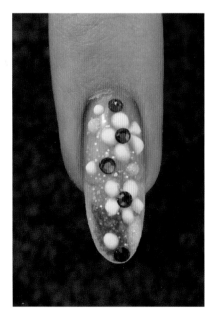

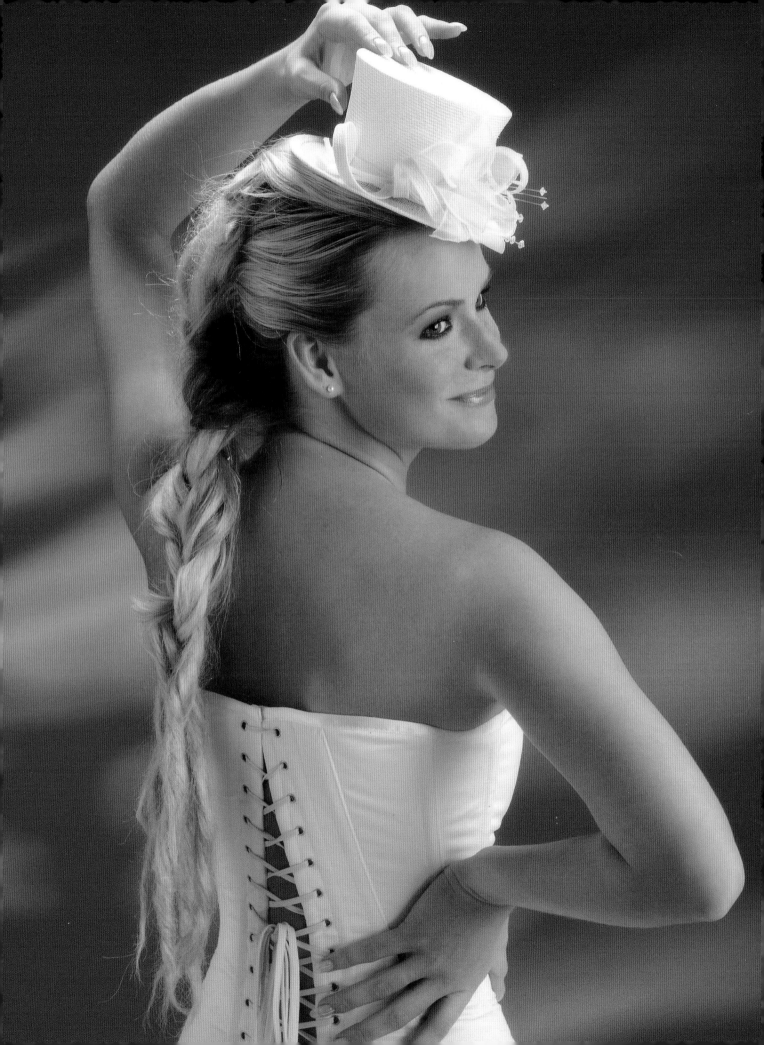

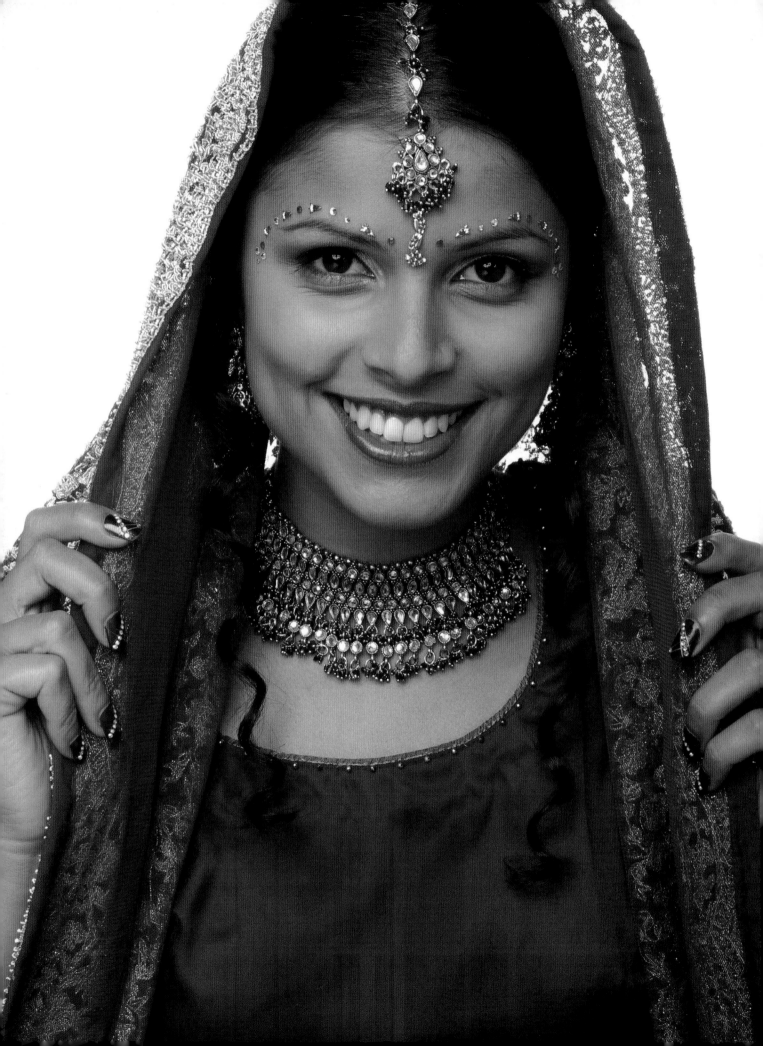

Asian bride

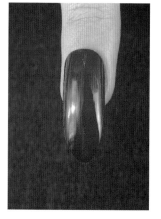

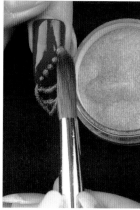

1 Shape and file nails to bride's requirements. Base coat with Stickey and then polish nails with Creative Moroccan Ruby Enamel. Use two coats of enamel.

2 Using a sculpting form make your own bhindi using Creative Metro Melting Pot Powder. Using Melting Pot Powder and Retention + apply small beads in a line from one corner of the nail up towards the cuticle. Ensure acrylic beads are not too wet, work dry.

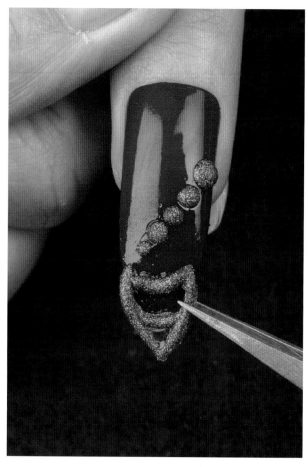

3 Ensure that the bhindi is placed on the tip. Apply with small beads of Gel Bond Adhesive.

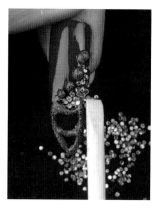

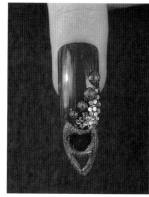

4 Apply small amount of Creative Super Shiney Top Coat to the area just above bhindi. Using gold flat stones fill in the area between dots and bhindi.

5 Ensure all flat stones are pressed firmly into position and then apply small amount of Super Shiney Top Coat.

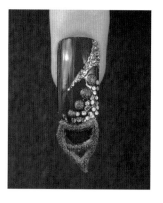

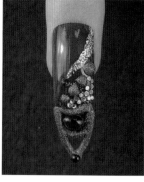

6 Using a small amount of gold glitter apply a stripe down the nail just above the gold dots.

7 Top coat with Creative Super Shiney. Take one large and one small red crystal and with Gel Bond apply in between bhindi and at the end of the glitter stripe.

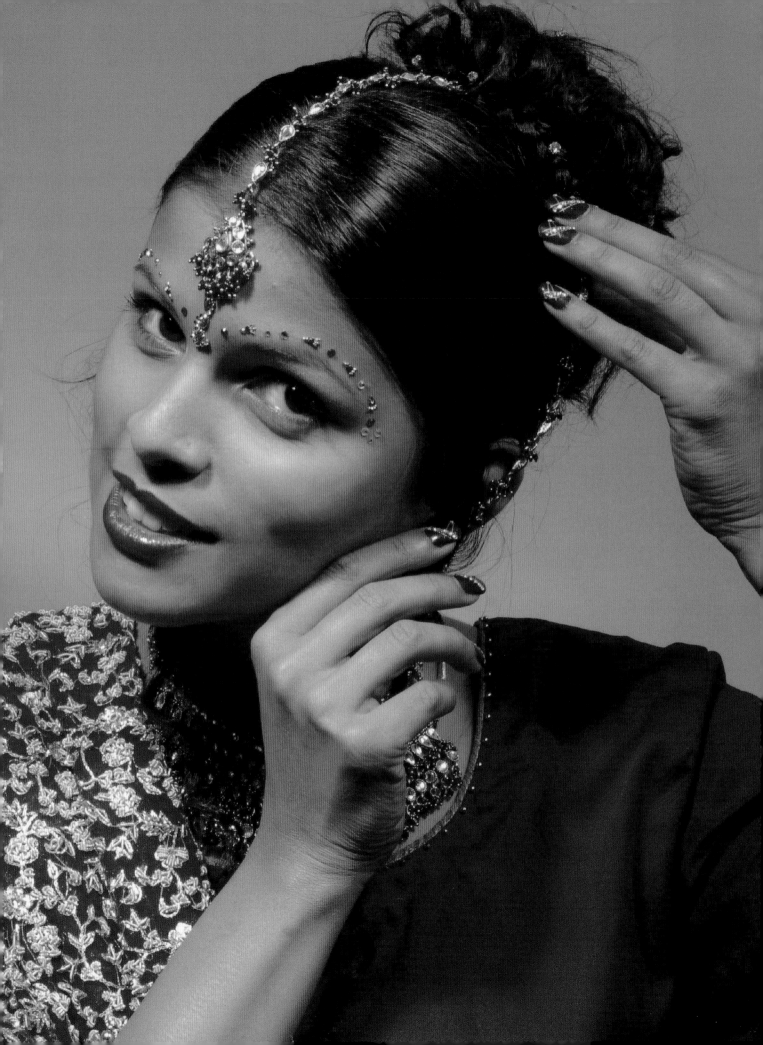

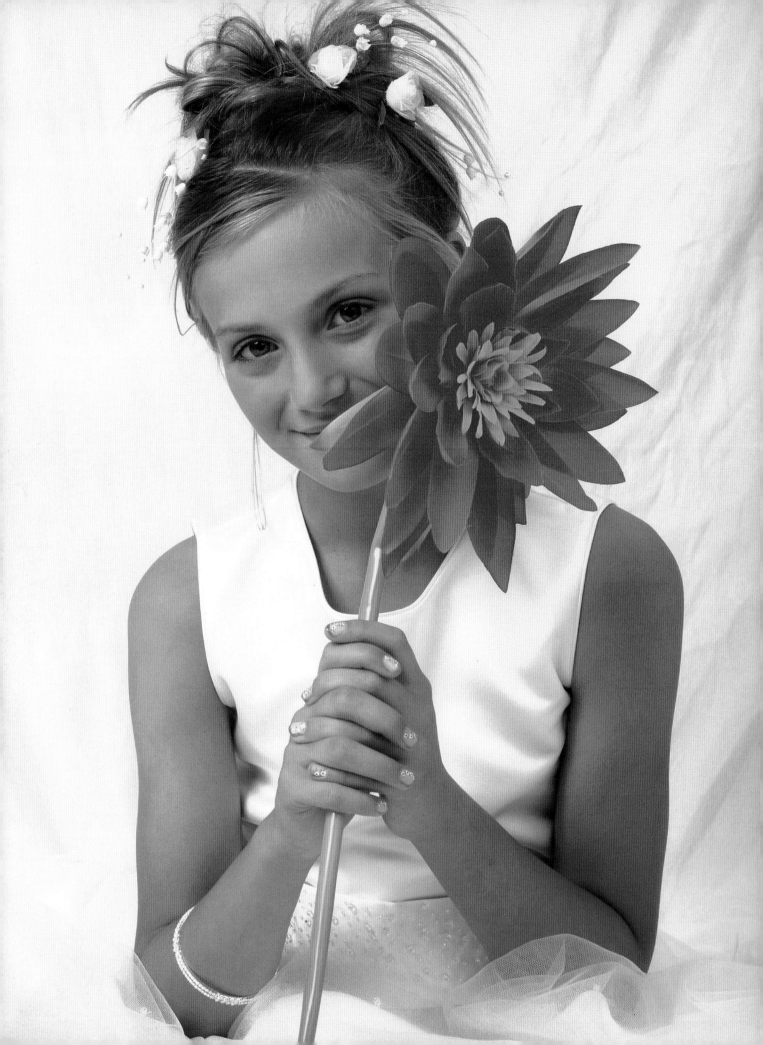

Bridesmaid

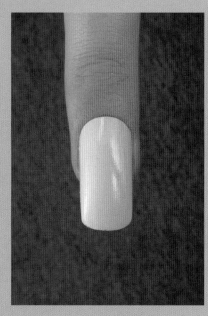

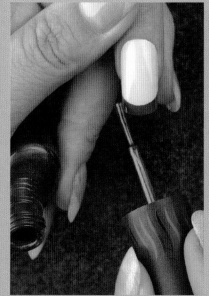

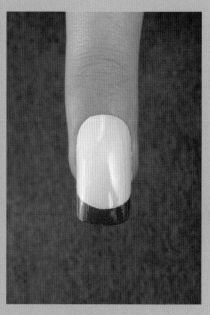

1 Base nails with Creative Stickey Base Coat. Paint with two coats of Creative Candied Violet Enamel.

2 Using Creative Plum Puckered Out Enamel apply to free edge creating a smile line.

3 If you need to, use a fine brush to neaten the line.

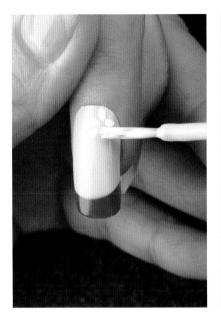

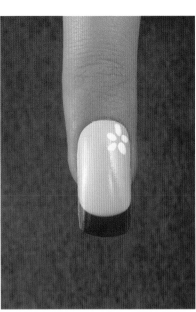

4 Apply small dots of Creative Cream Puff enamel to create petals.

5 Use five or six applications to create a flower.

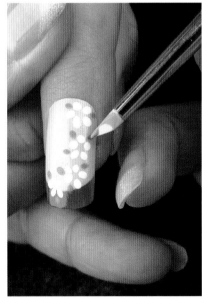

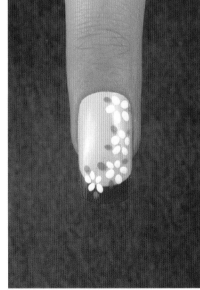

6 Using a colour shaper and some green paint apply a small leaf either side of each flower.

7 Flowers can either be positioned down the nail or across the smile line. Have some examples to show your clients.

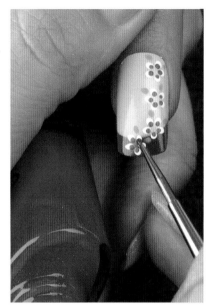 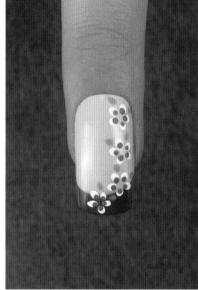 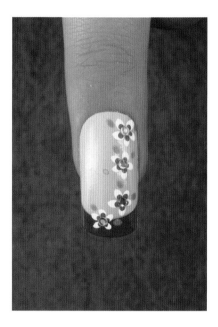

8 Using a dotting tool apply a small amount of Creative Candy Apple Enamel in the centre of each petal.

9 Adding another colour into the petals gives the flowers some dimension. Experiment with different colours.

10 Apply top coat and then using a dampened orange stick apply small yellow rhinestones as the centre piece of each flower. Ensure rhinestones are pressed into wet top coat for maximum adhesion.

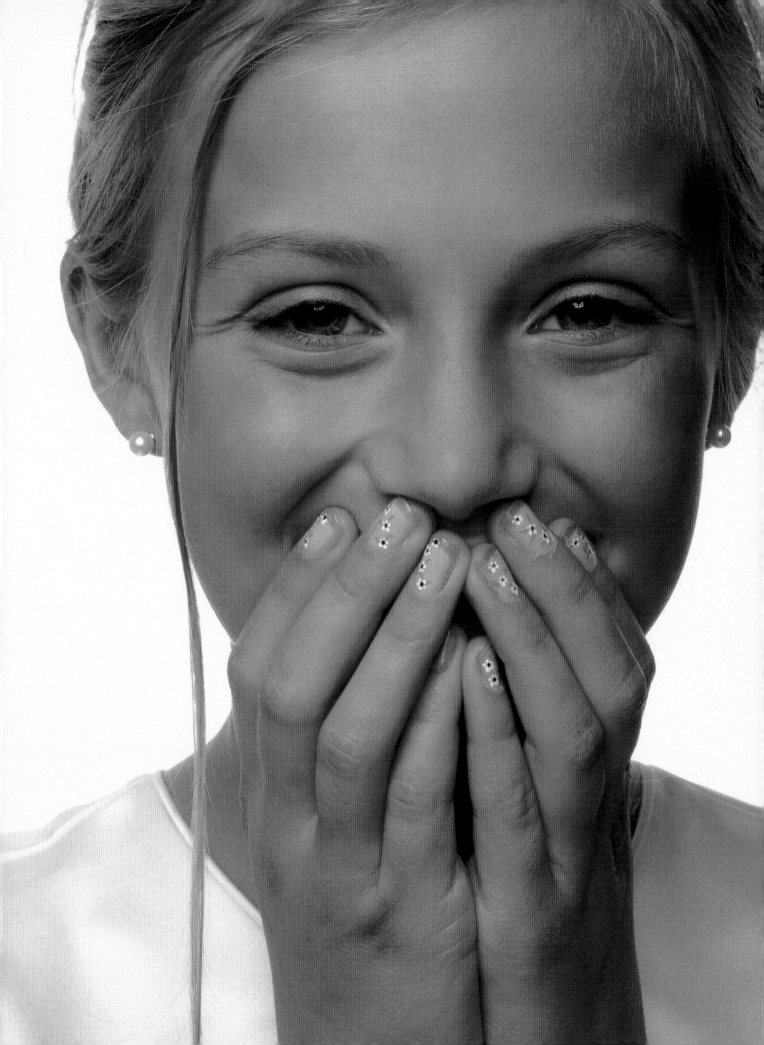

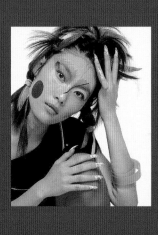
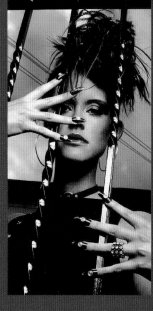
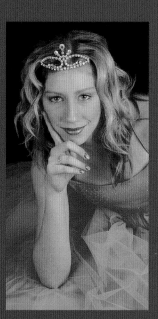

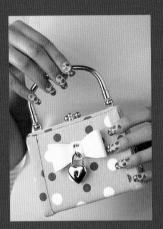

teenage

Sporty punk

Disco diva

Prom girl

Funky handbag

Come on England

Candy girl

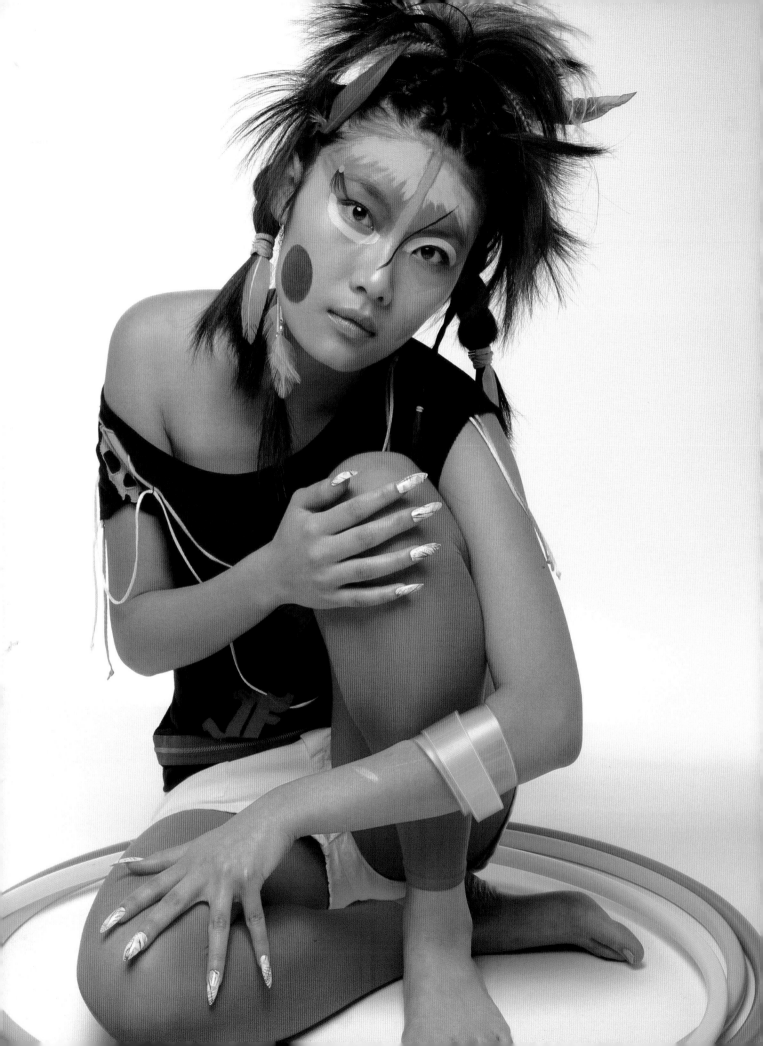

Sporty punk

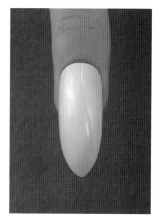 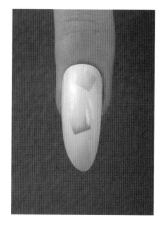 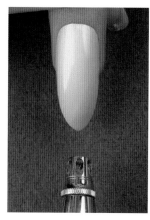 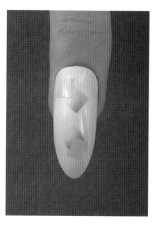

1 Apply a base coat to nails. With an airbrush spray Sudo light green over entire nail.

2 Using a slightly darker blue/green Sudo paint spray the tip of the nail to create a colour fade.

3 Hold a stencil gently on the nail and spray blue Sudo paint over three corners. Leaving one corner lighter than the others gives the illusion of 3D.

4 Using the same square stencil but now using an opaque peach Sudo colour spray over onto the two blue squares. You will need to use an opaque colour to block out the blue underneath.

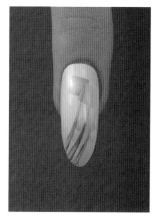 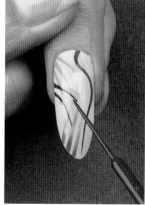 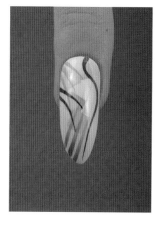 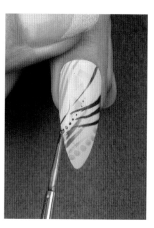

5 Take a striping brush and, using the same blue paint as for the squares, brush from the corner of the tip up into the centre of the nail.

6 Using the same striping brush but this time with yellow, orange and red paints brush the colour from sides to middle and from the top down to the free edge.

7 You can do many variations of this design using an exciting range of complementary colours. Do some designs in different colours to show your clients.

8 Using a dotting tool take a small amount of paint and dot from outer edge of nail into the centre following the lines. You will find the dots naturally get smaller as you have less paint on the tool.

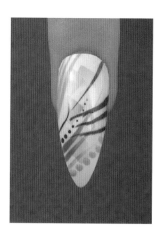

9 Once all the paint is dry use Creative Super Shiney Top Coat to give a glossy protective layer.

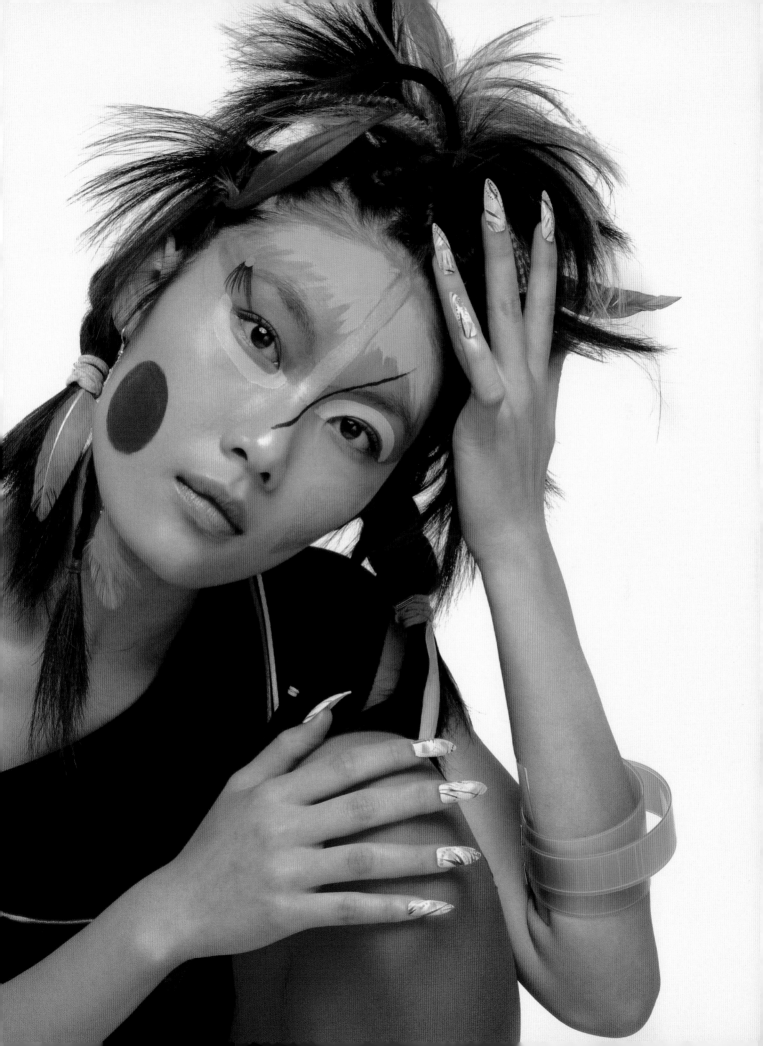

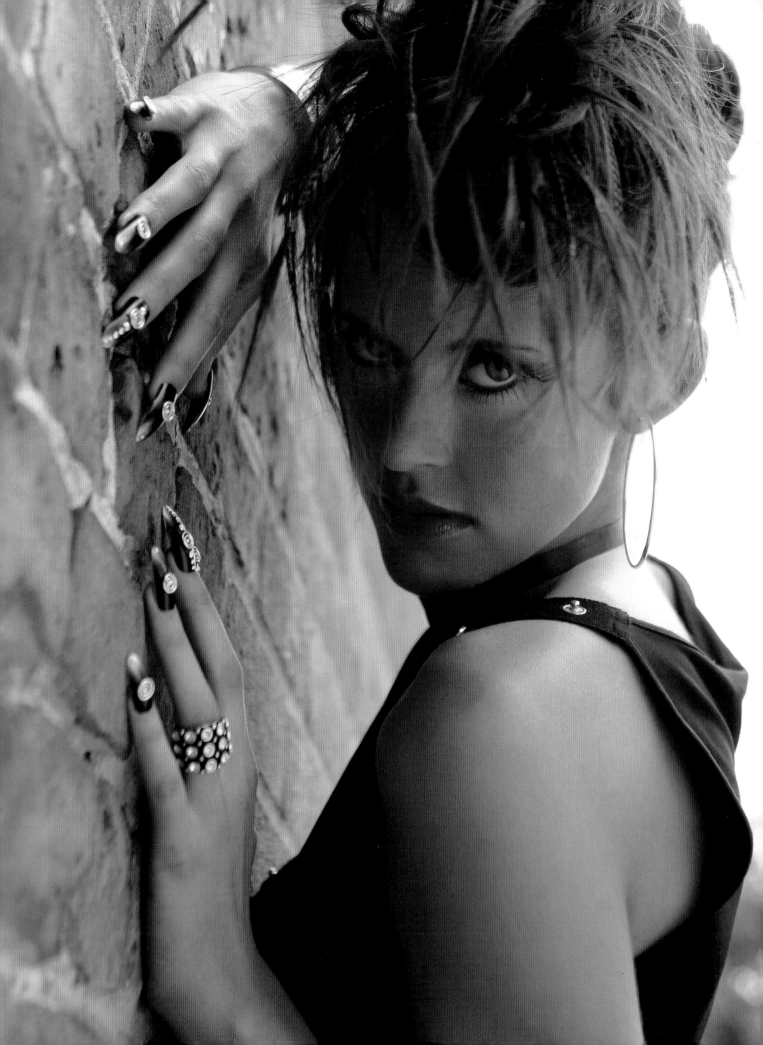

Disco diva

Disco diva

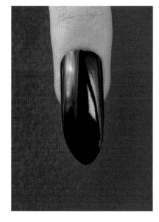

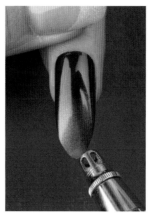

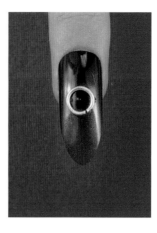

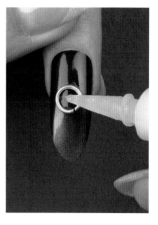

1 This design can also be easily achieved either with an airbrush or enamels. First apply your base coat and then either spray black opaque paint or use Creative Voodoo Enamel.

2 If using an airbrush spray Sudo silver paint onto the free edge of the nail. If using an enamel, polish with Creative Times Square at the free edge and blend up into the black.

3 Place two small beads of Gel Bond off centre on the nail and taking a silver ring with tweezers place it exactly in the centre of the nail.

4 Taking Gel Bond again place two small beads just inside the larger ring.

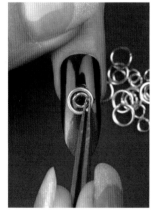

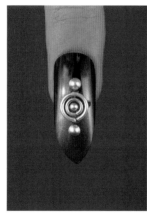

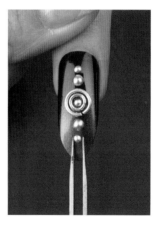

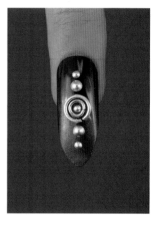

5 Taking a smaller silver ring with tweezers place in the centre of the larger ring.

6 Place small beads of Gel Bond Adhesive in the centre of the rings and at the top and bottom. With tweezers place hollow-backed silver studs on the adhesive.

7 Repeat process using slightly smaller studs.

8 Repeat process until studs are from top to bottom of nail.

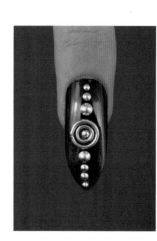

9 This design does look better when using different size studs and rings. Try out different variations.

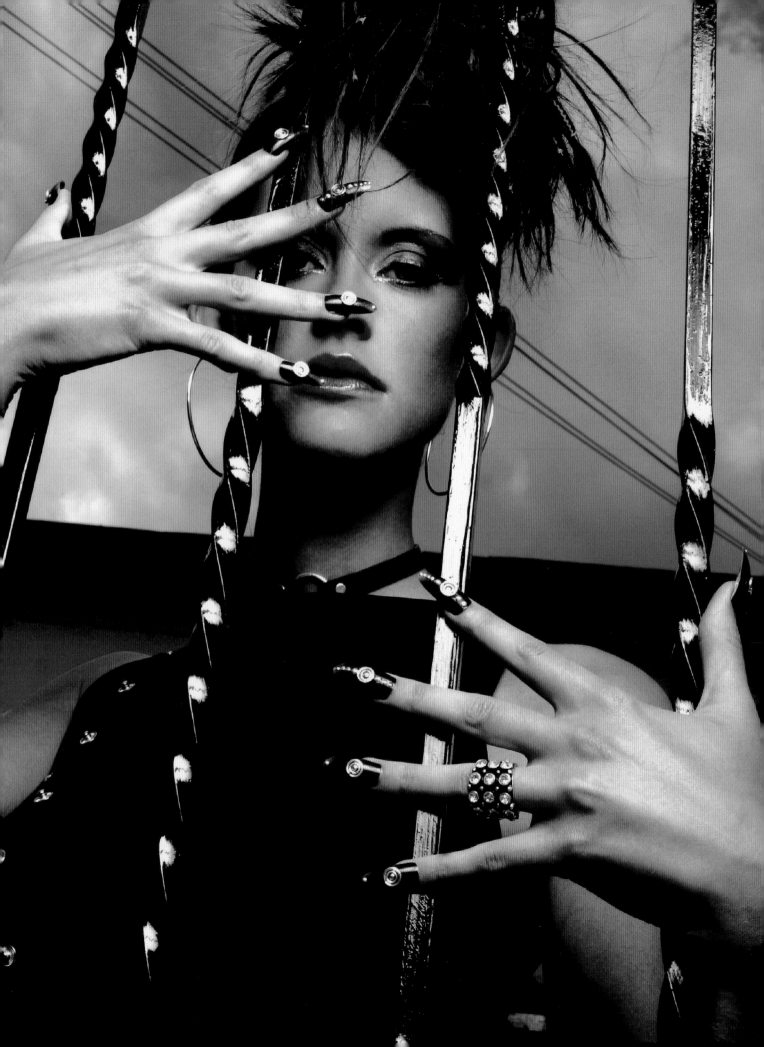

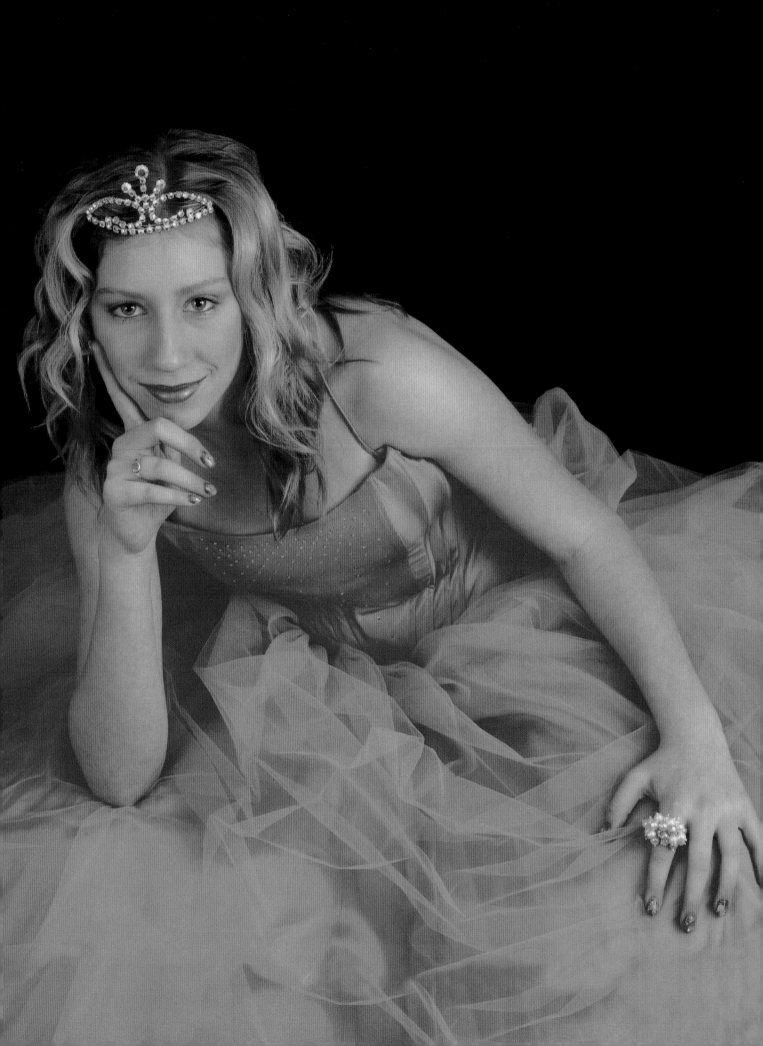

Prom girl

Prom girl

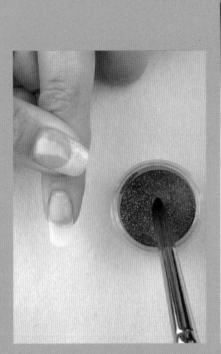

1 Apply, blend to natural nail and shape Creative Velocity Tips.

2 Take a bead of Creative Spanish Tile Mosaic Powder, dip it into red glitter to form a bead and place onto the free edge of the tip.

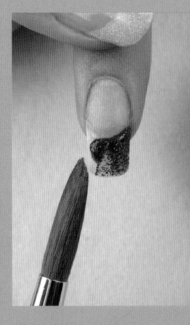

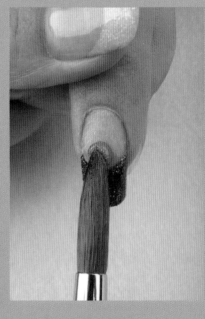

3 Press the bead into place creating a smile line.

4 Take a bead of Creative Perfect Clear Powder, dip it into a baby pink glitter and apply to middle of the nail. Press and smooth into shape.

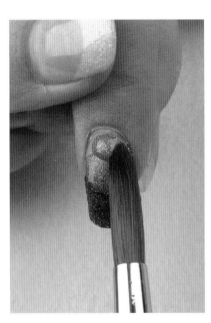

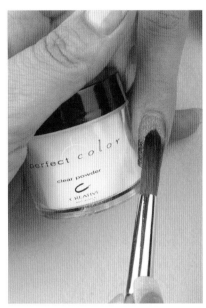

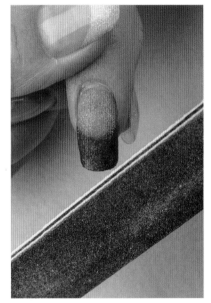

5 Apply second bead in the cuticle area being careful not to touch surrounding soft tissue.

6 Apply a thin coat of Creative Perfect Clear Powder over the whole nail.

7 File and buff to shape. Be careful not to buff through the clear powder as this may affect the colour of the glitter.

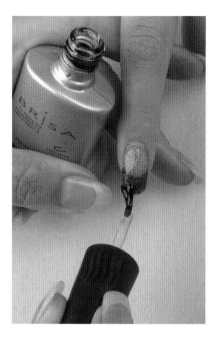

8 Apply some Scrubfresh and then apply one thin coat of Creative Brisa Finishing Gloss UV Gel.

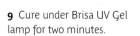

9 Cure under Brisa UV Gel lamp for two minutes.

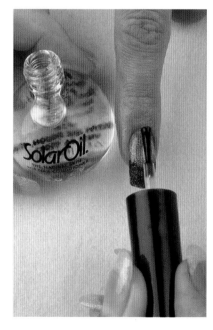

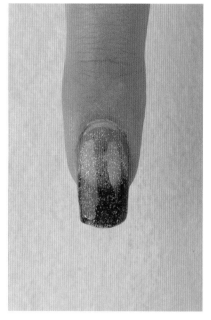

10 When cured wipe off sticky layer with Scrubfresh and apply Solar Oil.

11 Creative Mosaic Powders can be mixed with one another to create many beautiful colours. Try variations of this design. It is effective yet simple. The finished acrylic nails can have extra decoration added by hand painting and adding some rhinestones.

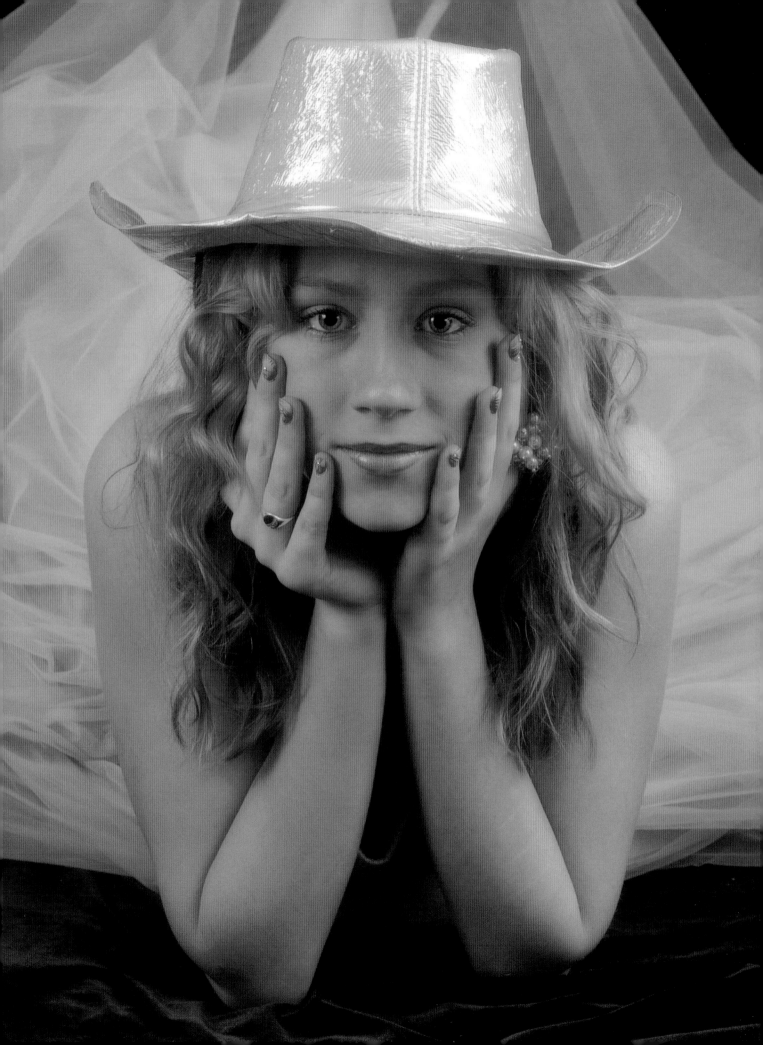

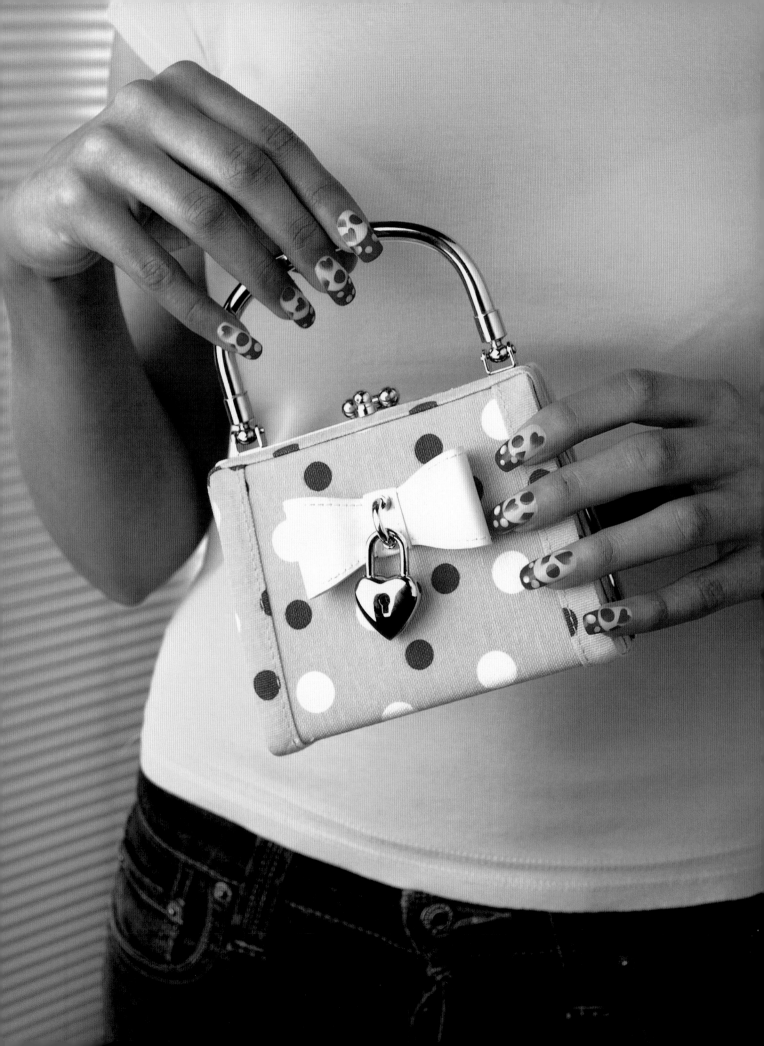

Funky
handbag

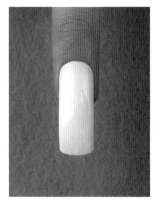

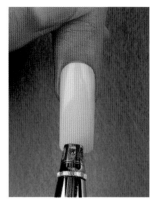

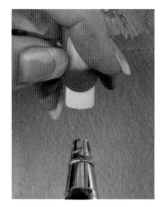

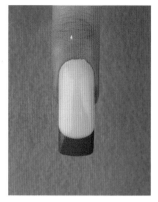

1 This design can be achieved using either an airbrush or by hand painting. Airbrush is quicker and easier. Base coat nails and then spray with Sudo opaque white.

2 Spay with bright yellow Sudo opaque paint.

3 Holding a stencil across the free edge, spray red opaque Sudo paint to achieve a French polish.

4 This can be achieved with Creative nail enamels – Sugar Rush, Hot Pop Yellow and Cream Puff.

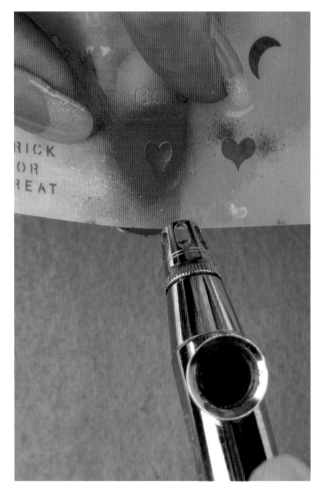

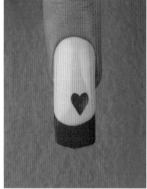

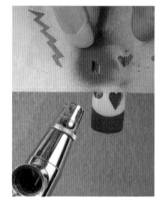

6 Leaving a shadow at one side of the heart gives the illusion of 3D.

7 Spray again through stencil randomly over the entire yellow area using different shapes.

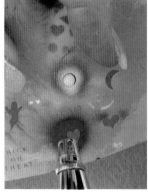

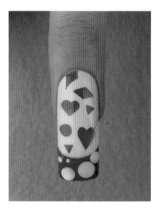

5 Holding a stencil, spray through with red opaque Sudo paint onto the yellow in the shapes that match the handbag.

8 Taking opaque white Sudo paint, spray through a stencil with circles on the red dot area.

9 Once the deired look has been achieved and the paint is dry, seal and then top coat. Remember that any handbag can be matched in some way and it is a great way of accessorising.

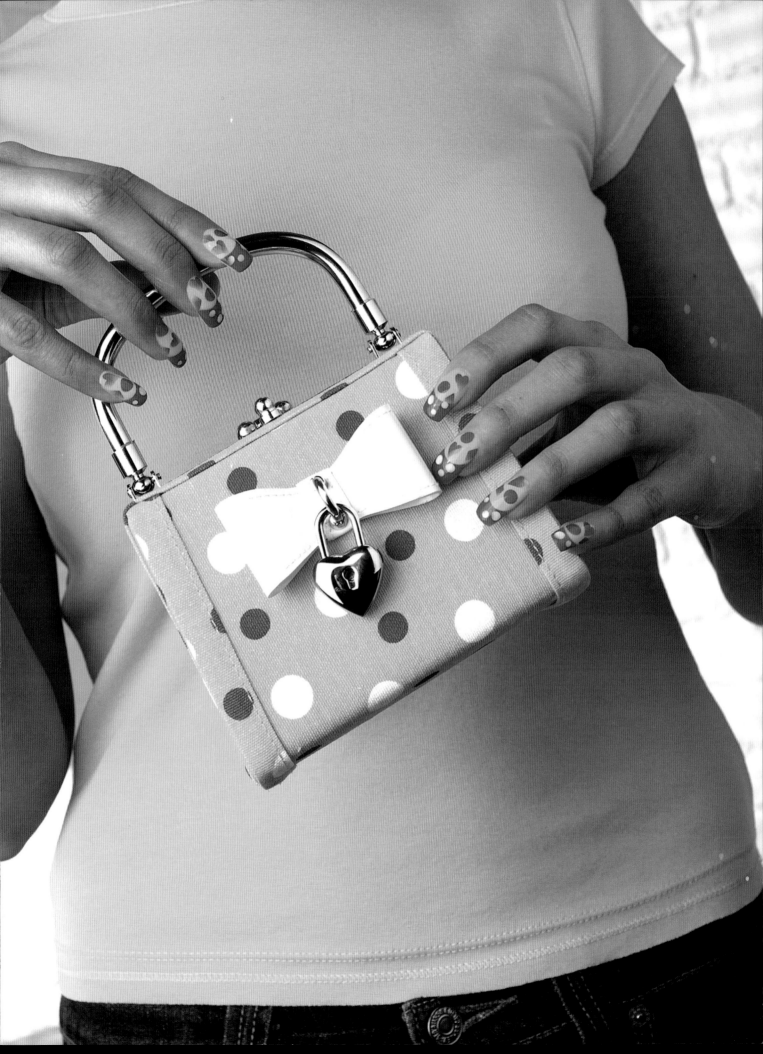

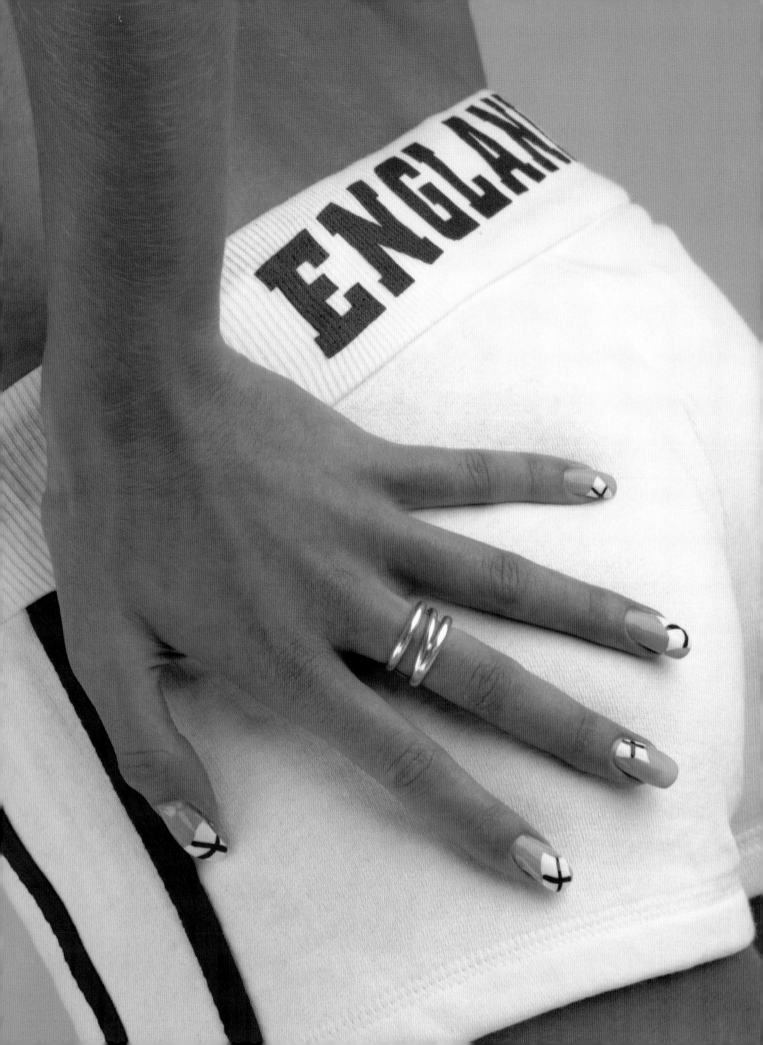

Come on England

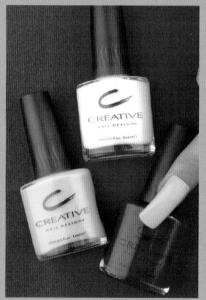

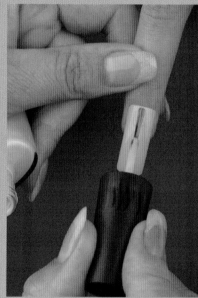

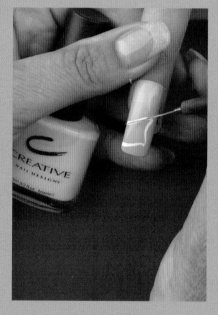

1 Every year nail technicians get asked to paint the national flag on clients' nails because of various sporting events. Here is a slightly different angle on the English flag.

2 Base coat all ten nails with Stickey. Then, using two coats of Creative Hot Pop Blue Nail Enamel, polish nails.

3 Once enamel is dry using Creative Cream Puff Enamel and a small striping brush draw an outline of a flag on the end of the nail. Give the lines some movement as if the flag is flying.

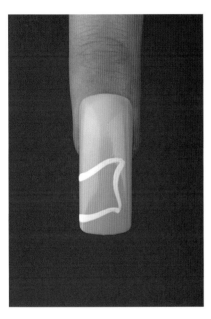 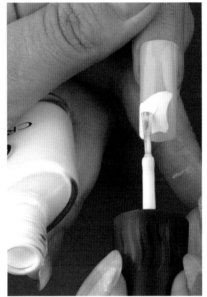 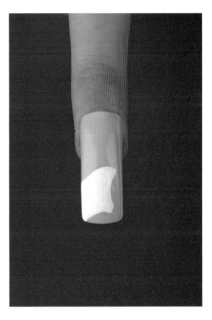

4 You can see from the main picture the various positions that you may put the flags in on the nails. Try to do a different position on each nail: it makes it more interesting.

5 Fill in between the lines with Cream Puff Enamel.

6 Do not worry if the white enamel is slightly bumpy as the top coat should cover this.

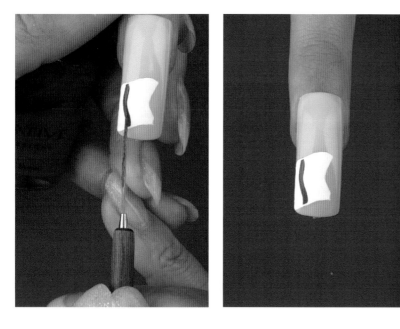

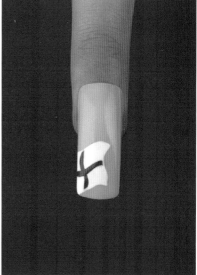

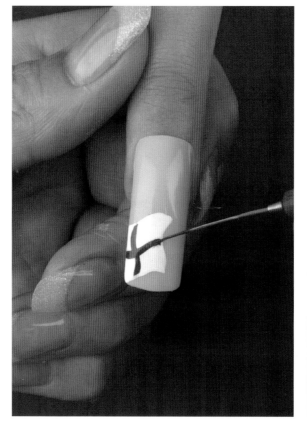

7 Using the small striping brush and Creative Company Red Enamel draw a line down the flag just slightly off centre and with a slight wave to it.

8 Drawing lines just off centre gives the illusion of the flag flying which is heightened by the slight wave in the centre.

9 Using the same technique draw a red line across the flag.

10 Tidy up if needed with a small detail brush and top coat when paint is dry. Top coat with Super Shiney.

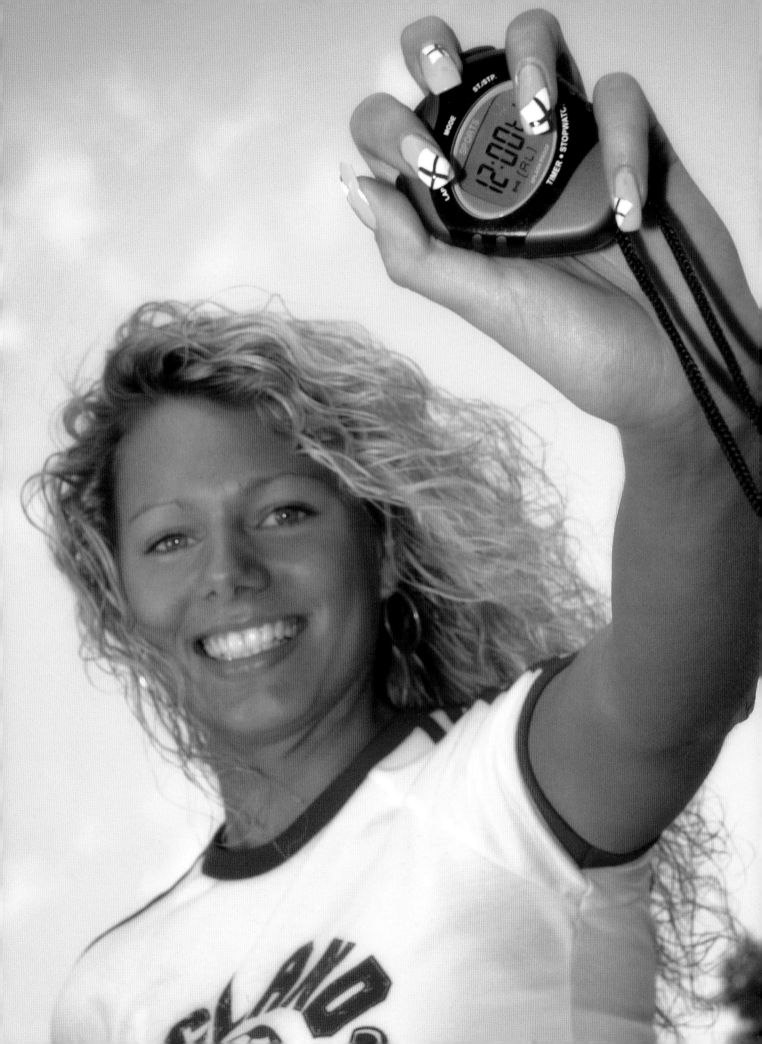

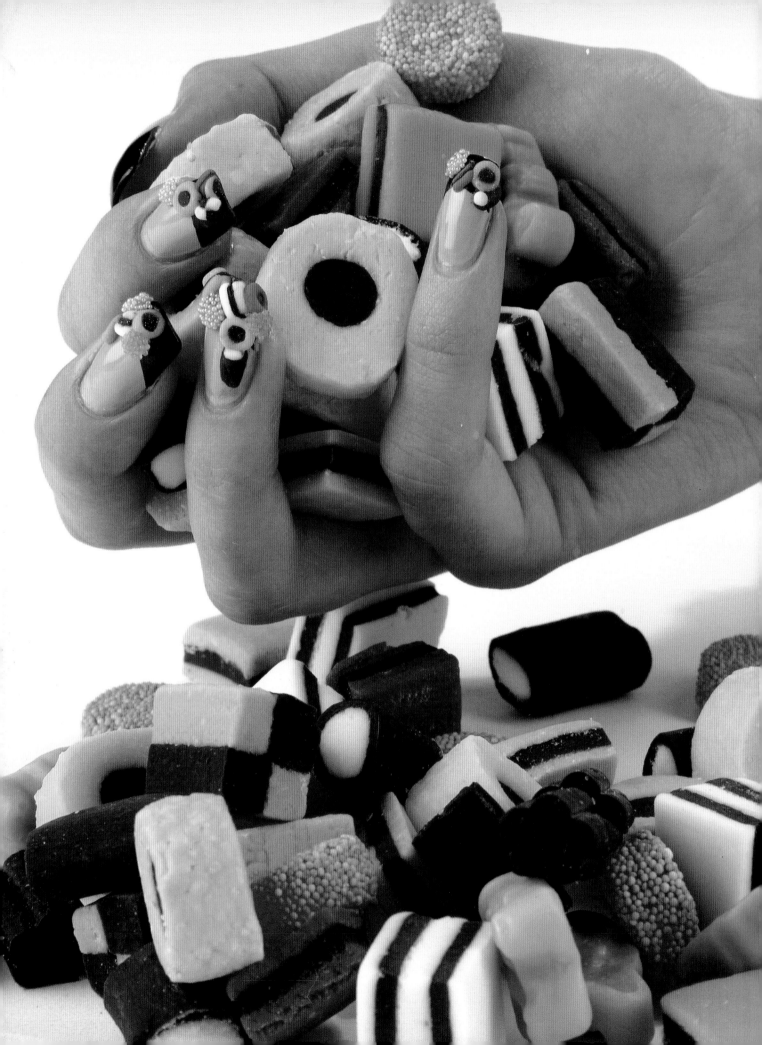

Candy girl

Candy girl

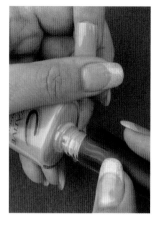

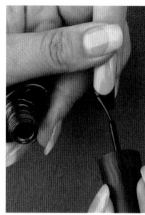

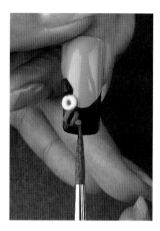

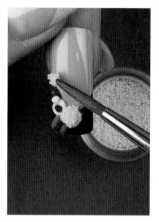

1 Base nails with Sticky Base Coat. Apply two coats of Creative Grapeade Enamel.

2 Use Creative Voodoo Enamel polish on the free edge, creating a French polish.

3 Taking Creative Terra Cotta Mosaic Powder and Retention + put small bead onto nail and shape into separate two squares. Fill in with Creative Black Powder.

4 Taking a small bead of Creative Perfect Clear Powder dip it into small decorative beads to create a look-a-like sweet. Place onto the nail next to other sweets and allow to settle.

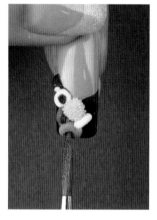

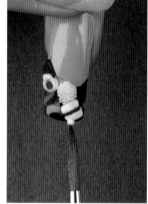

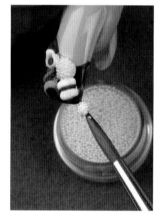

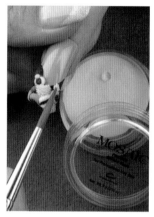

5 Take up a small bead of Creative Quartz Crystal Mosaic Powder and press onto the free edge of the nail. Hold brush in the centre of the bead to create a hole. Fill with Creative Black Powder.

6 Using Creative Perfect White Powder create two oblong shapes and fill centre with Creative Black Powder.

7 Using Creative Perfect Clear Powder create a bead and dip into pink decorative beads and apply to the edge of the nail next to last sweet.

8 Take a small bead of Creative Golden Glass Mosaic Powder and apply to the edge of the nail just above the pink sweet. Use brush to create a hole and fill with a small bead of Creative Black Powder.

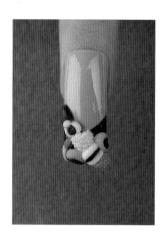

9 This design can be changed to suit any type of sweet. It looks great on Creative Clear Tips. Experiment with your techniques on sculpting forms before working on clients.

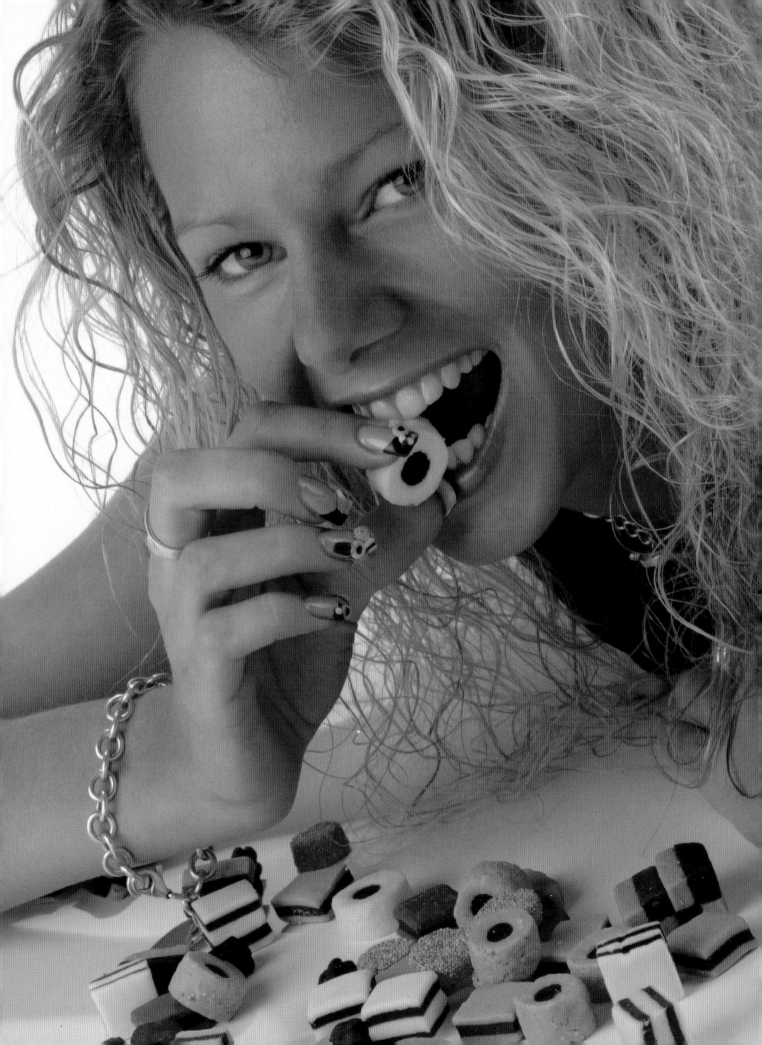

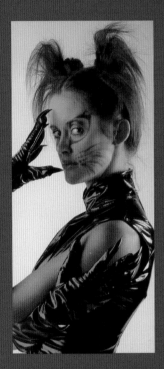

fancy dress

Flower girl

Cabaret

Cat woman

Moulin Rouge

Alien

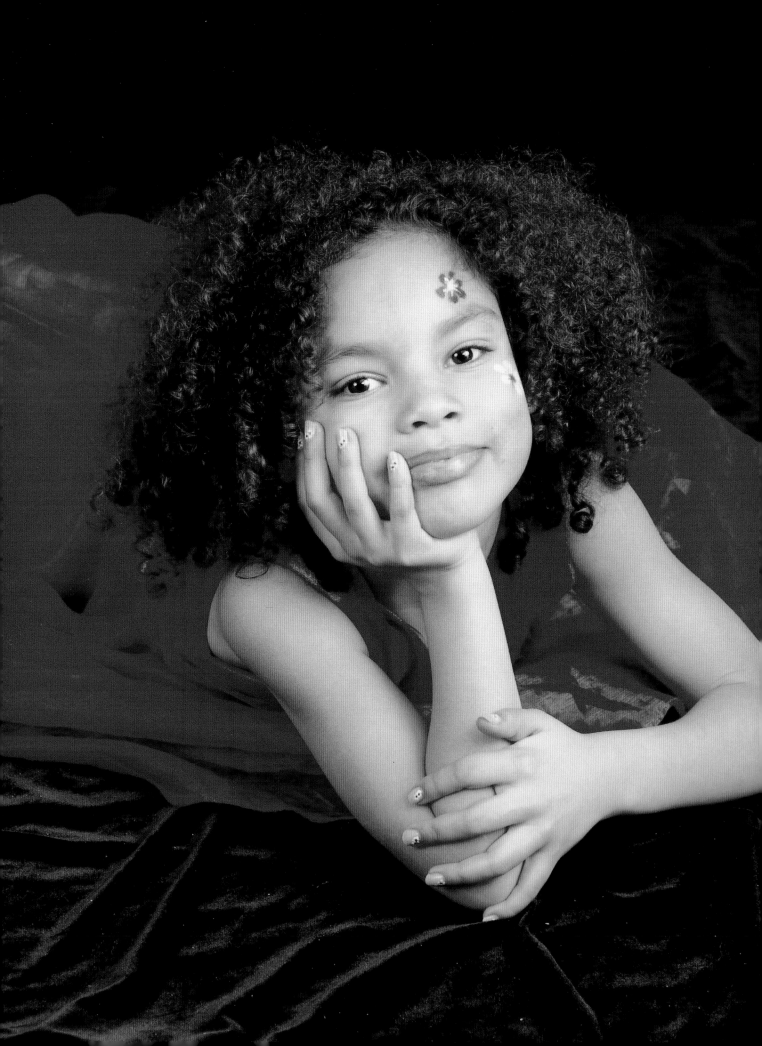

Flower girl

Flower girl

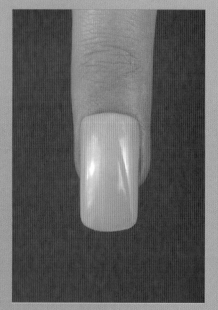

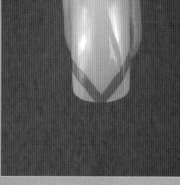

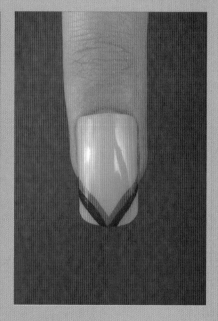

1 Apply Stickey Base Coat. Polish nails with two coats of Creative Hot Pop Yellow Enamel.

2 Take a striping brush and Creative Hot Pop Orange Enamel and draw two French chevron lines down into the tip of the nail.

3 Repeat the same technique with the striping brush, using Creative Candy Apple underneath the orange line.

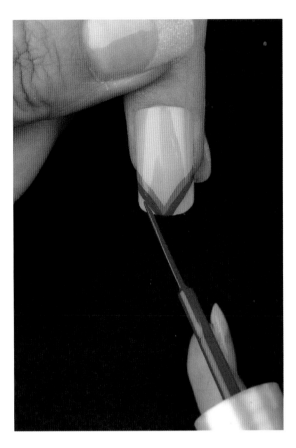

4 A striping brush will mean thinner and straighter lines than those you can make with an enamel brush. It is also easier to correct with this type of brush if you are working on more intricate designs.

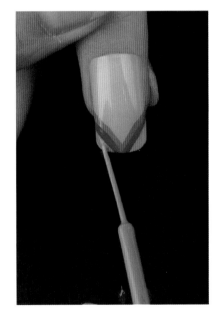

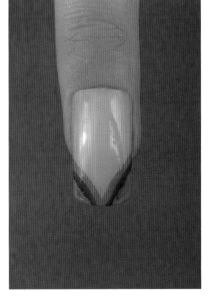

5 With the same striping brush draw a line of Creative Hot Pop Blue Enamel along the bottom of the red line.

6 Use the enamel brush to fill in the blue to the corners of the nail.

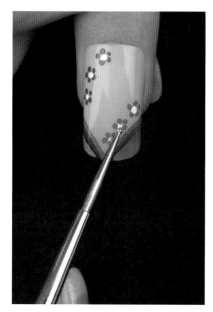

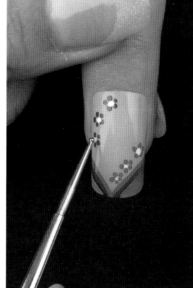

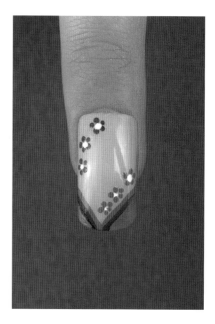

7 Using a dotting tool use Creative Hot Pop Orange Enamel to create small daisies along the orange line.

8 Repeat process with Creative Candy Apple Enamel along the other side of the nail towards the cuticle.

9 Use dotting tool to fill in the centre of each flower with Creative Cream Puff Enamel. Once polish is dry top coat with Creative Super Shiney.

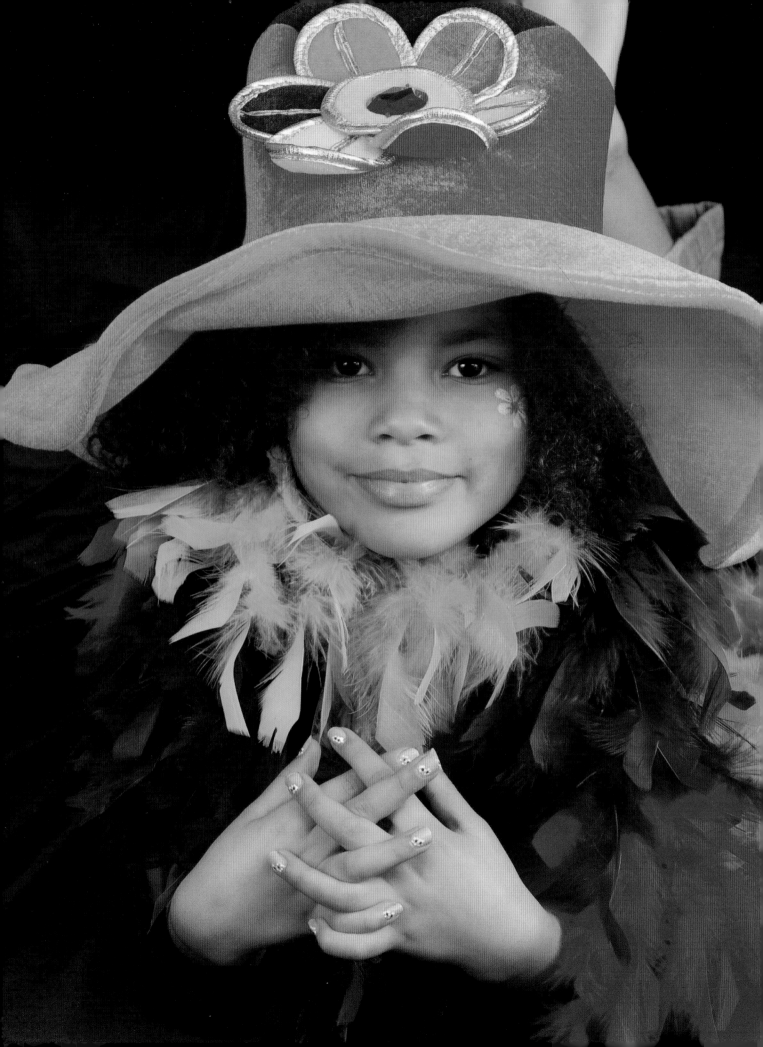

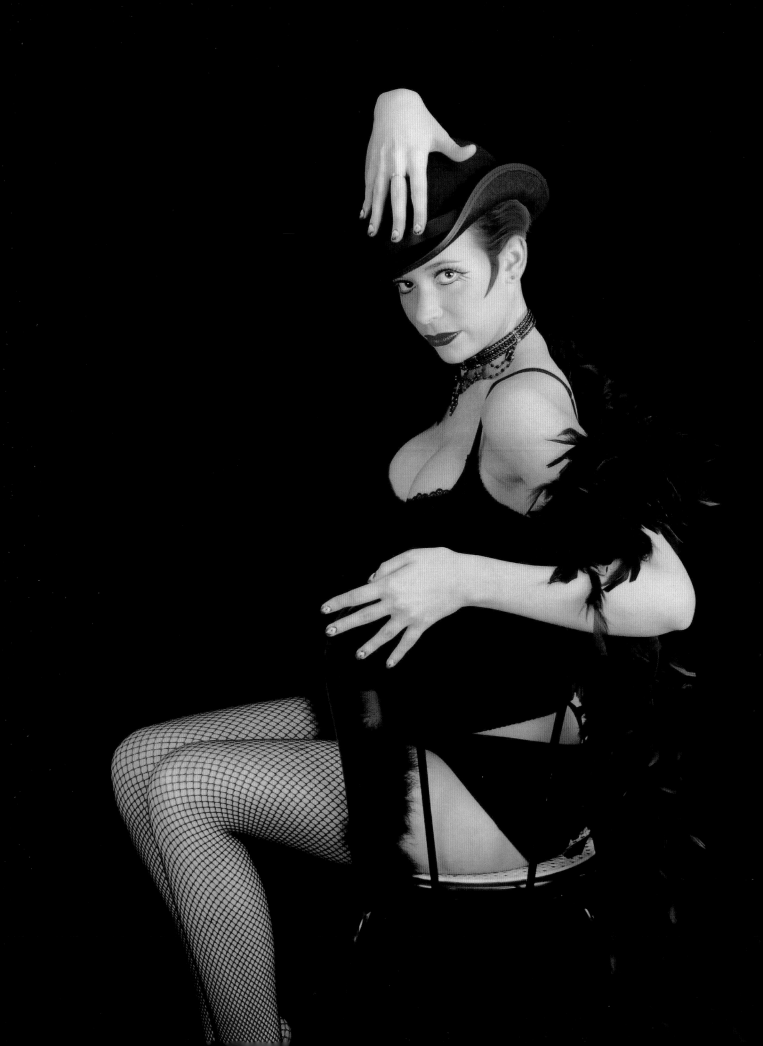

Cabaret

Cabaret

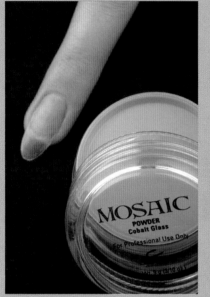

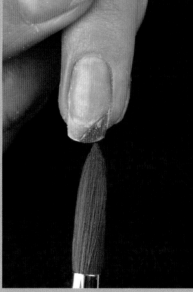

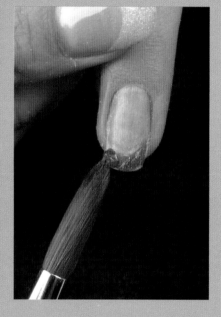

1 Apply, cut and blend to natural nail a Creative Clear Tip. Apply Scrubfresh to eliminate any oil and bacteria.

2 Apply Creative Cobalt Glass Mosaic Powder to one side of the tip and press into a triangle shape into corner.

3 Apply a second bead of Cobalt Glass and form the same shape on the other side of the tip.

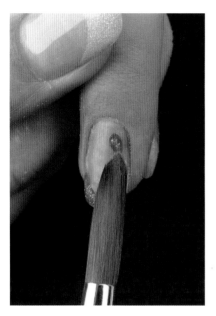

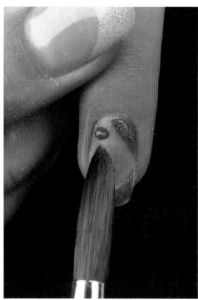

4 Put a small bead of Creative Quartz Crystal Mosaic Powder on top of nail near cuticle area and repeat the same shape as Cobalt Glass in one corner.

5 Repeat the same shape with Quartz Crystal on the other side of the nail.

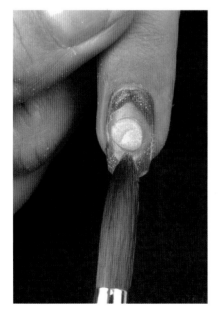

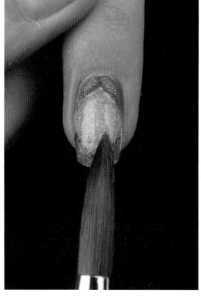

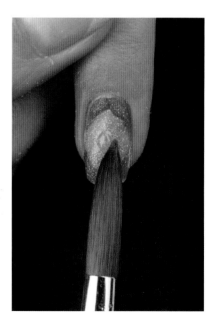

6 Apply a slightly larger bead of Creative Glimmer powder to the middle of the nail.

7 Press into shape without going over onto the other two colours.

8 Take a very small bead of Blue Cobalt and apply to the centre of the nail. Shape into a diagonal square. Keep shape in place with brush until product is almost set.

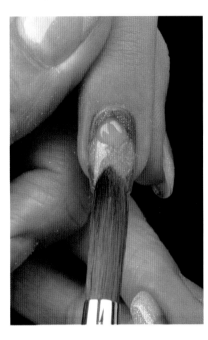

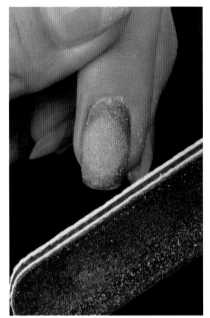

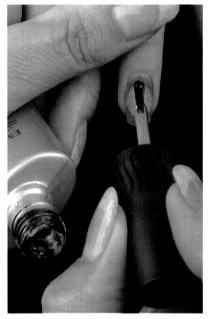

9 Apply thin layer of Creative Perfect Clear Powder over entire design.

10 File and buff. Clean off any dust with Scrubfresh.

11 Apply a thin layer of Creative Brisa Finishing Gloss and cure under Brisa UV lamp for two minutes.

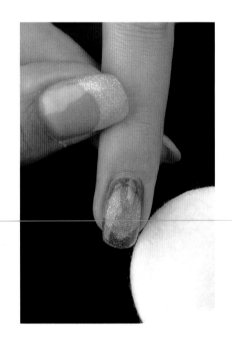

12 Wipe sticky residue away with Scrubfresh and apply a small amount of Solar Oil.

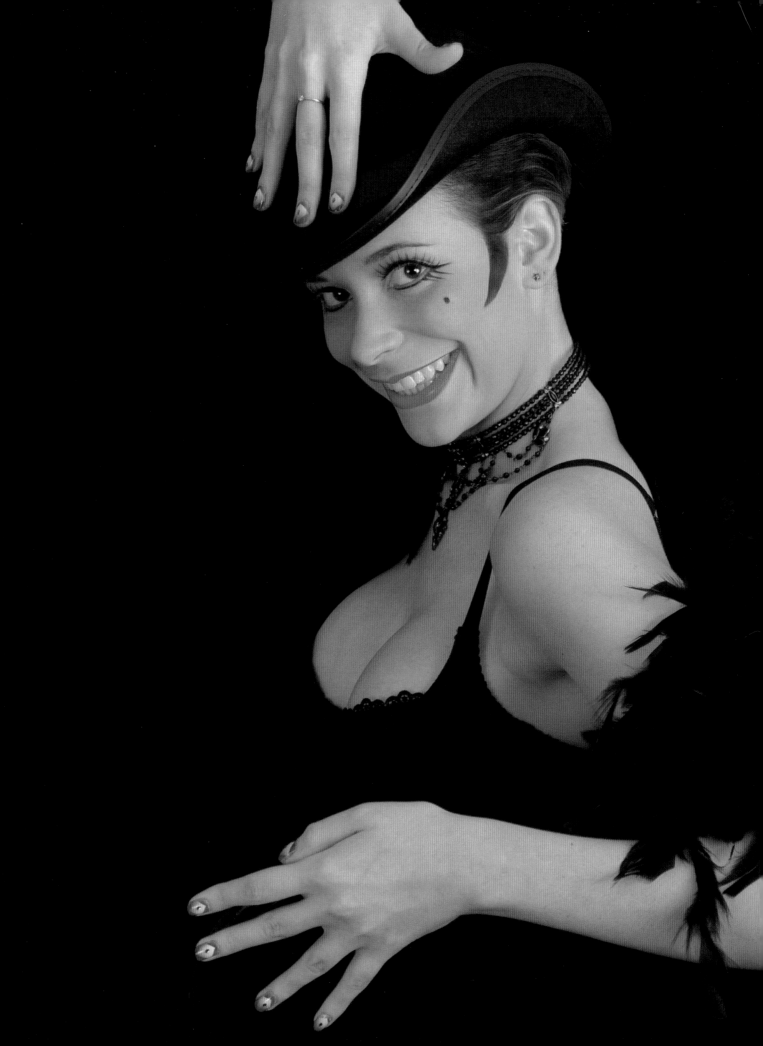

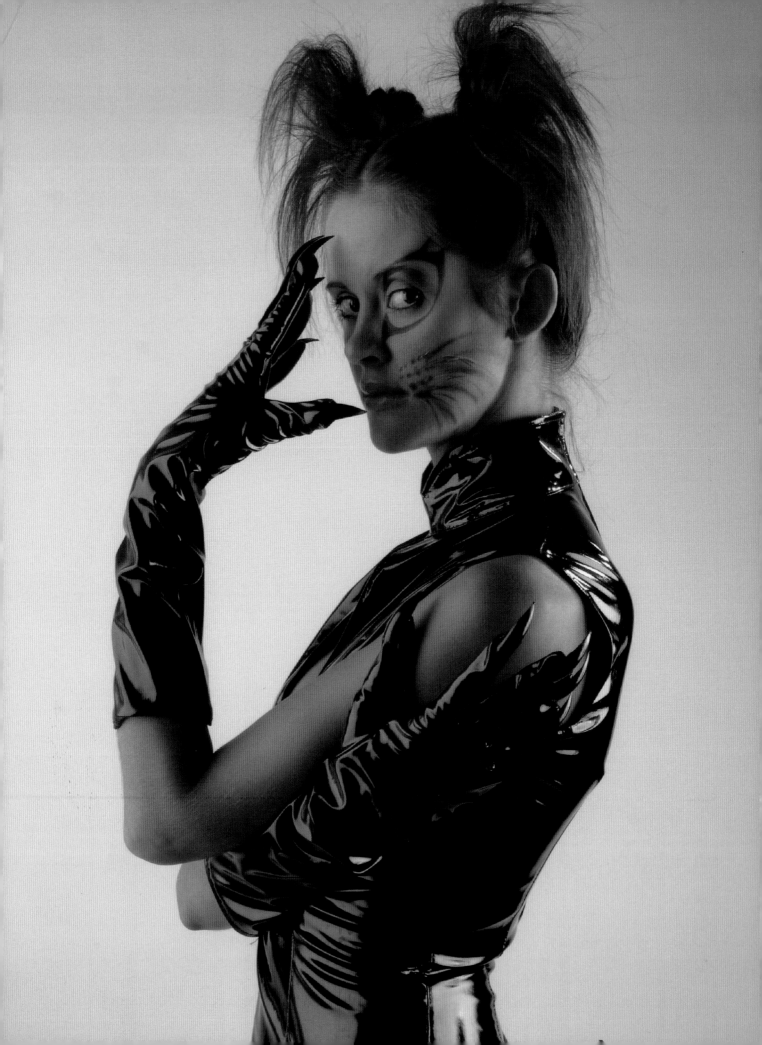

Cat woman

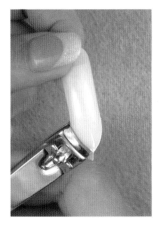 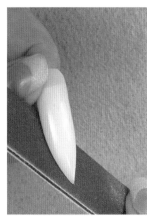 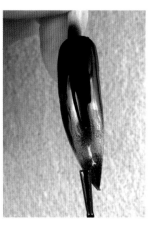 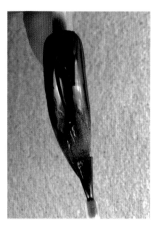

1 Take a long curve KISS tip and cut into either side to create a deep "V".

2 Finish shaping with a file to give a really neat point.

3 Apply Stickey Base Coat and then two coats of Creative Voodoo Enamel.

4 For effect Creative Enamel can be used on the end to give a colour fade. Then apply Super Shiny Top Coat.

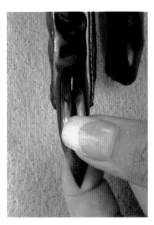 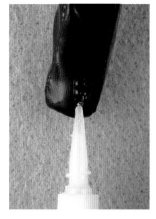

5 Take a pair of black PVC gloves and find someone to wear them for a minute whilst you apply the tips or wear them yourself.

6 Apply Gel Bond Adhesive to the tip of each finger of the glove.

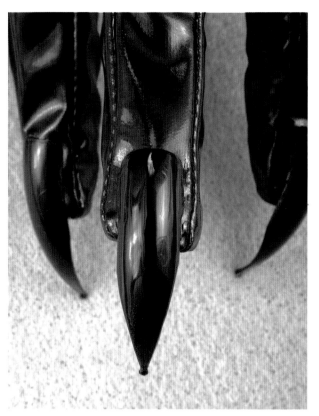

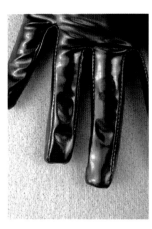 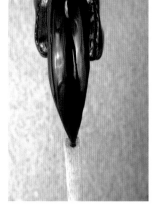

7 Press tip into place and hold firmly for at least twenty seconds each tip. The tip should mould into the shape of the fingernail underneath.

8 Apply another coat of Super Shiney and apply with a dampened orange stick a dark red rhinestone to the end of the tip.

9 Allow to dry. If you are going to a fancy dress and want to be outrageous but it is impractical to wear long nails, use this theme and make gloves instead.

They are much easier to remove and can be kept for future use.

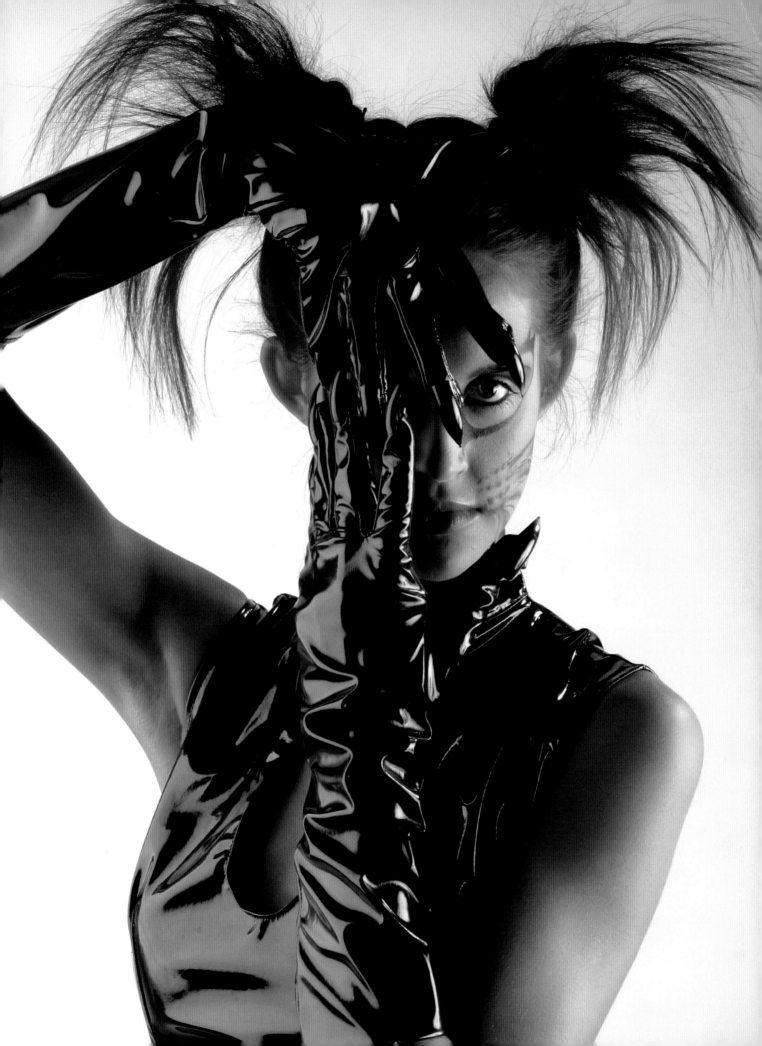

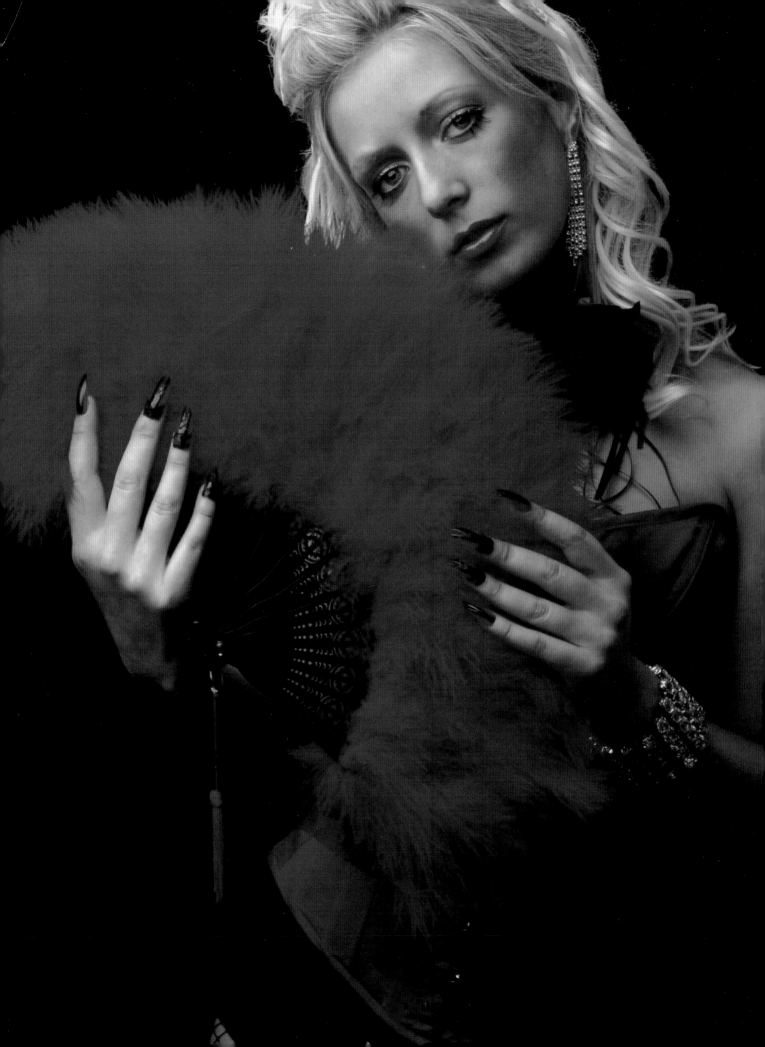

Moulin Rouge

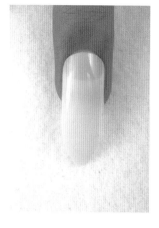 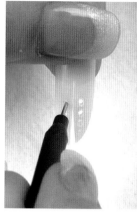 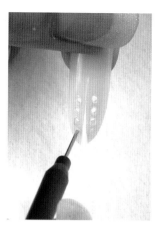 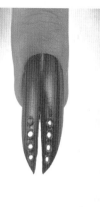

1 It is advisable to do this design on tips before applying them to the nails because of the cutting and drilling involved. Cut and shape tip.

2 Cut with sharp scissors up the centre of the nail to about half way. Cut a thin slice again giving you a slight parting in the nail.

3 Drill four small holes in either side of the split, just slightly away from the side.

4 Base coat the nail with Stickey. Allow to dry and polish the nails with two coats of Creative Fiesta Enamel.

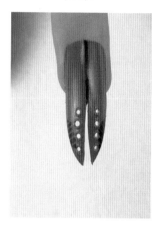 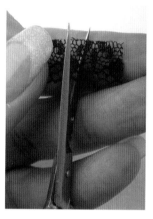

5 With a small striping brush and Creative Voodoo Enamel paint a line from the cuticle to the split in the nail and around six small lines at the side of the holes.

6 Take a piece of small lace and cut to suit shape of top half of nail.

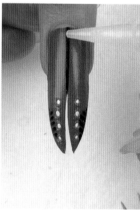 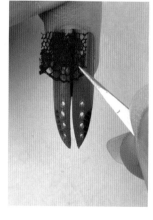

7 Apply small beads of Gel Bond to edges of nail where lace will sit.

8 Apply lace with tweezers to the top half of the nail and hold down in place until dry.

9 Using a needle weave black cotton thread through the holes to make a corset effect. Tie small knot in the back of

the cotton and cut thread off. You can match any corset with this nail using different colours, lace and thread.

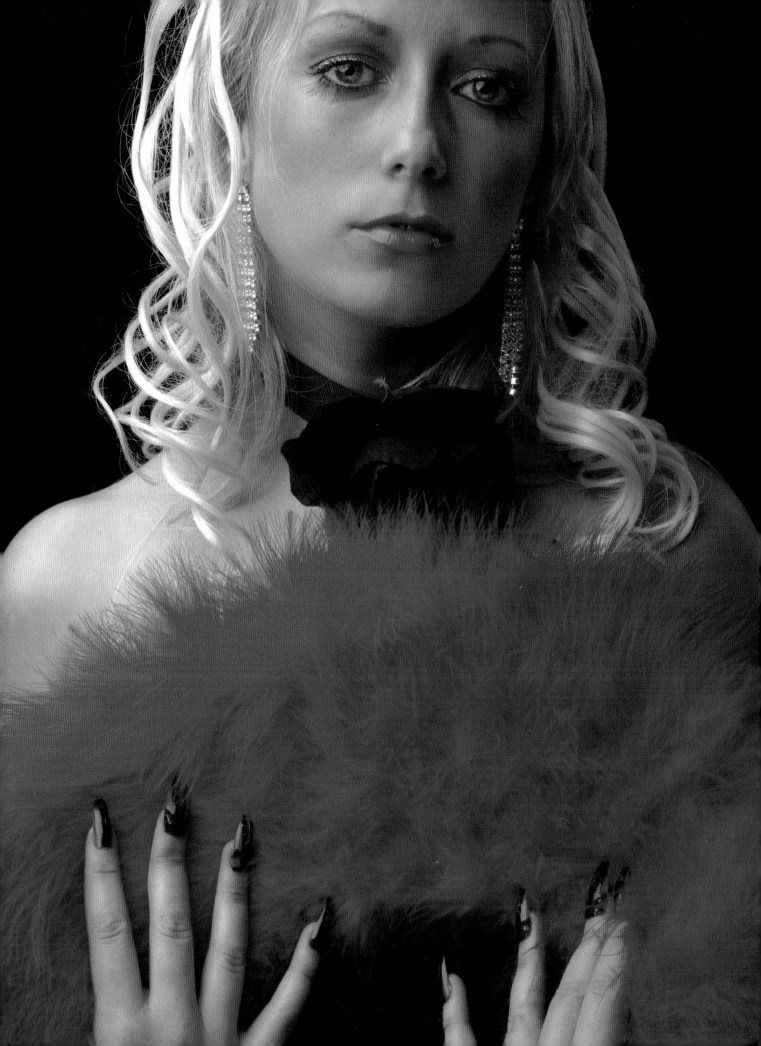

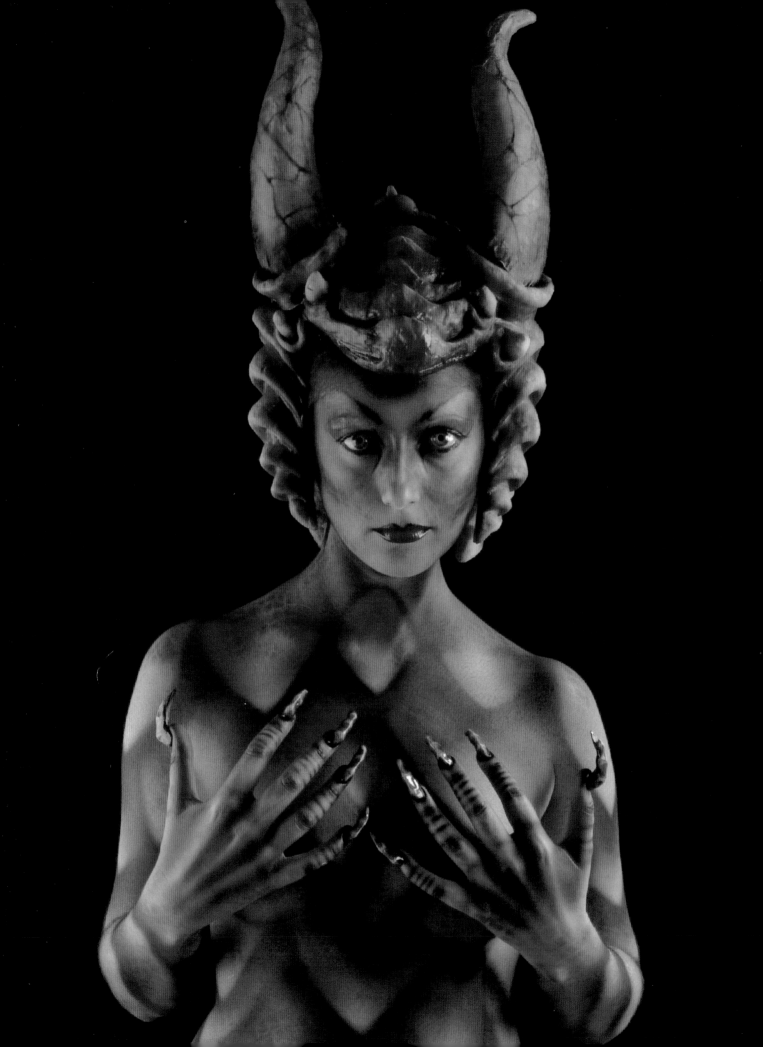

Alien

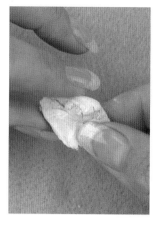

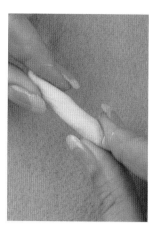

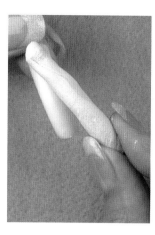

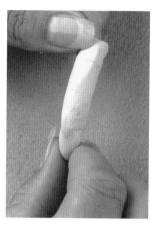

1 Take some modelling clay and start moulding into shape.

2 Press into shape; it should be slightly longer than your tip.

3 Apply small amounts of Gel Bond Adhesive to the tip and press clay onto it covering the whole tip with the clay.

4 Allow the clay to adhere to the tip before you start moulding the shape.

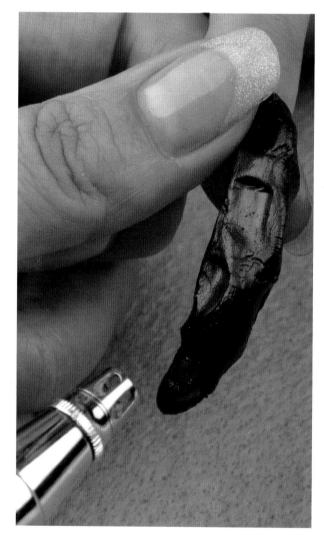

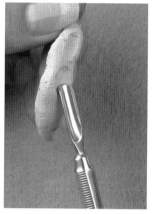

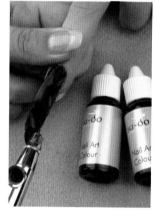

5 Using an appropriate tool start shaping the clay into a claw.

6 Spray with an airgun the shaped alien nails with black Sudo opaque paint.

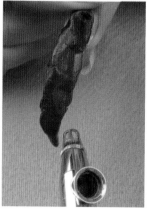

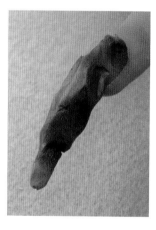

7 Then spray with Sudo gold Paint into the holes made by the tool.

8 Using a light Sudo brown paint start to contour the shape of the nail.

9 Use a dark yellow paint to highlight the nail. Finish with a top coat and your alien nails are ready. See Hen Night nails in Bridal Section (p.53) for safe application method.

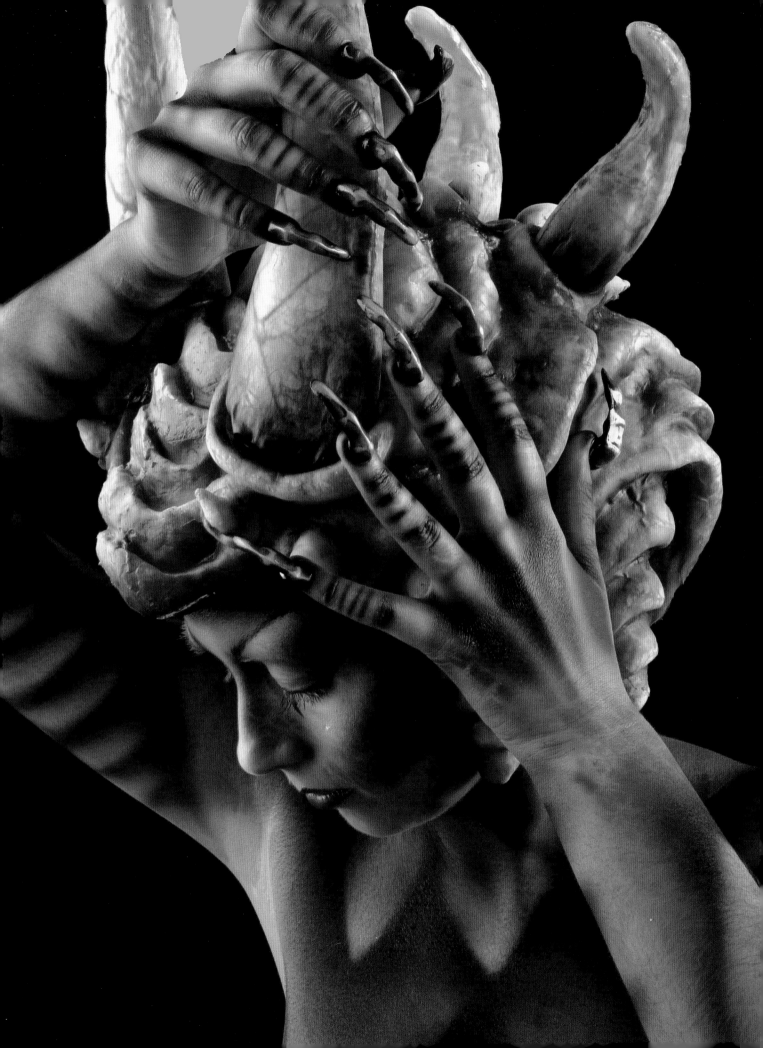

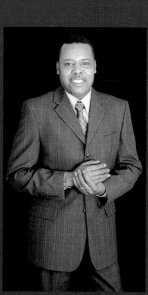
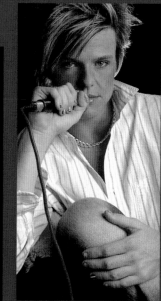

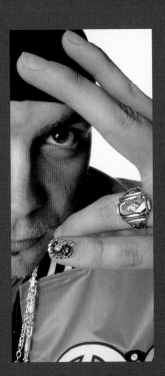

men

Weatherman

Boy band

Rap artist

Soul man

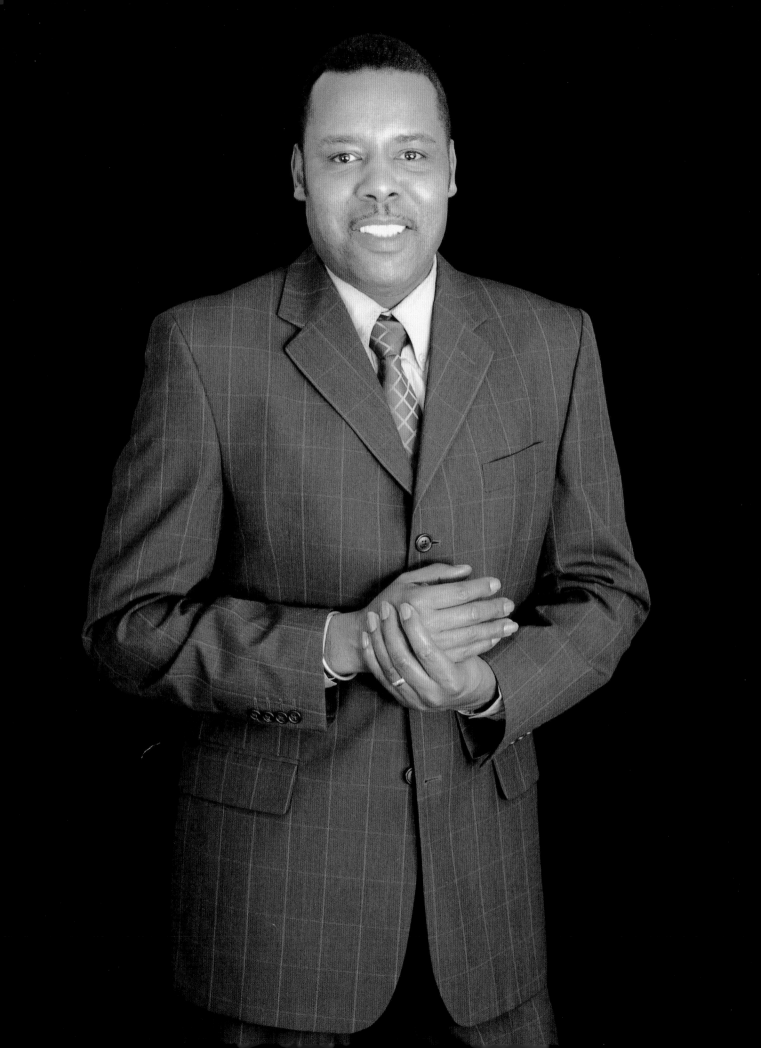

Weatherman

Weatherman

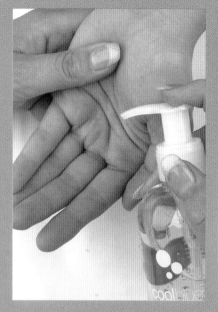

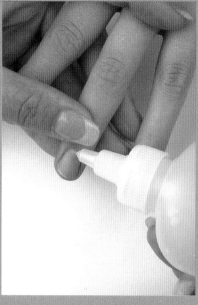

1 Manicures are for everyone, even Everton Fox who is a real BBC Weatherman. This is one of the quickest manicures with great results. Firstly sanitise the hands of you and your clients with Cool Blue.

2 Apply Creative Cuticle Remover and push cuticle back with a cuticle pusher. Spray hands with water and wash away the remover. Dry with towel.

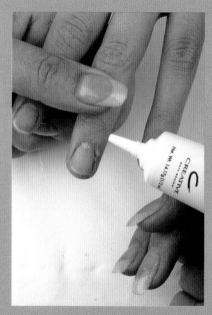

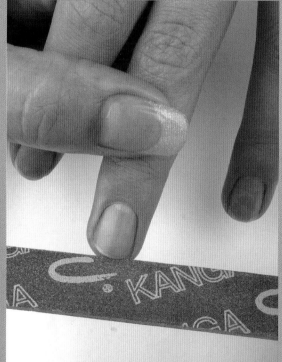

3 Apply SolarBalm cuticle treatment and massage into cuticles.

4 File free edge of nails with a Creative Kanga Board.

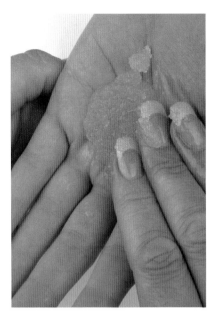

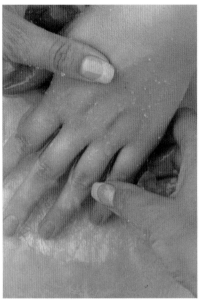

5 Take a small spoonful of Solar Manicure and massage into the hands up to the wrist.

6 With a warm bowl of water wash excess Solar Manicure off of the hands.

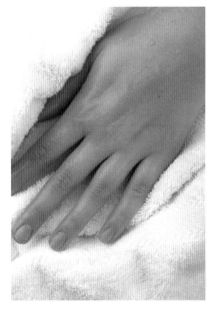

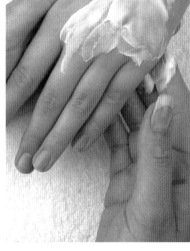

7 Dry hands thoroughly with clean dry towel.

8 Apply small amount of Solar Butter and perform hand and wrist massage.

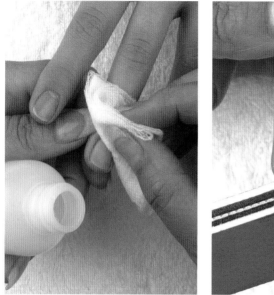

9 Squeak nails with Scrubfresh to eliminate any cream and oil on the nail plate.

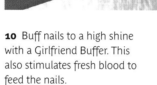

10 Buff nails to a high shine with a Girlfriend Buffer. This also stimulates fresh blood to feed the nails.

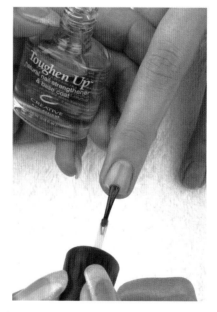

11 Apply a coat of Creative Toughen Up which is a nail strengthener.

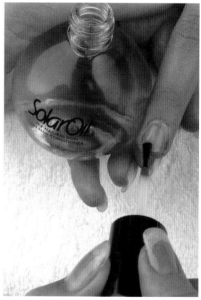

12 Finish with a small amount of Solar Oil and massage into nails.

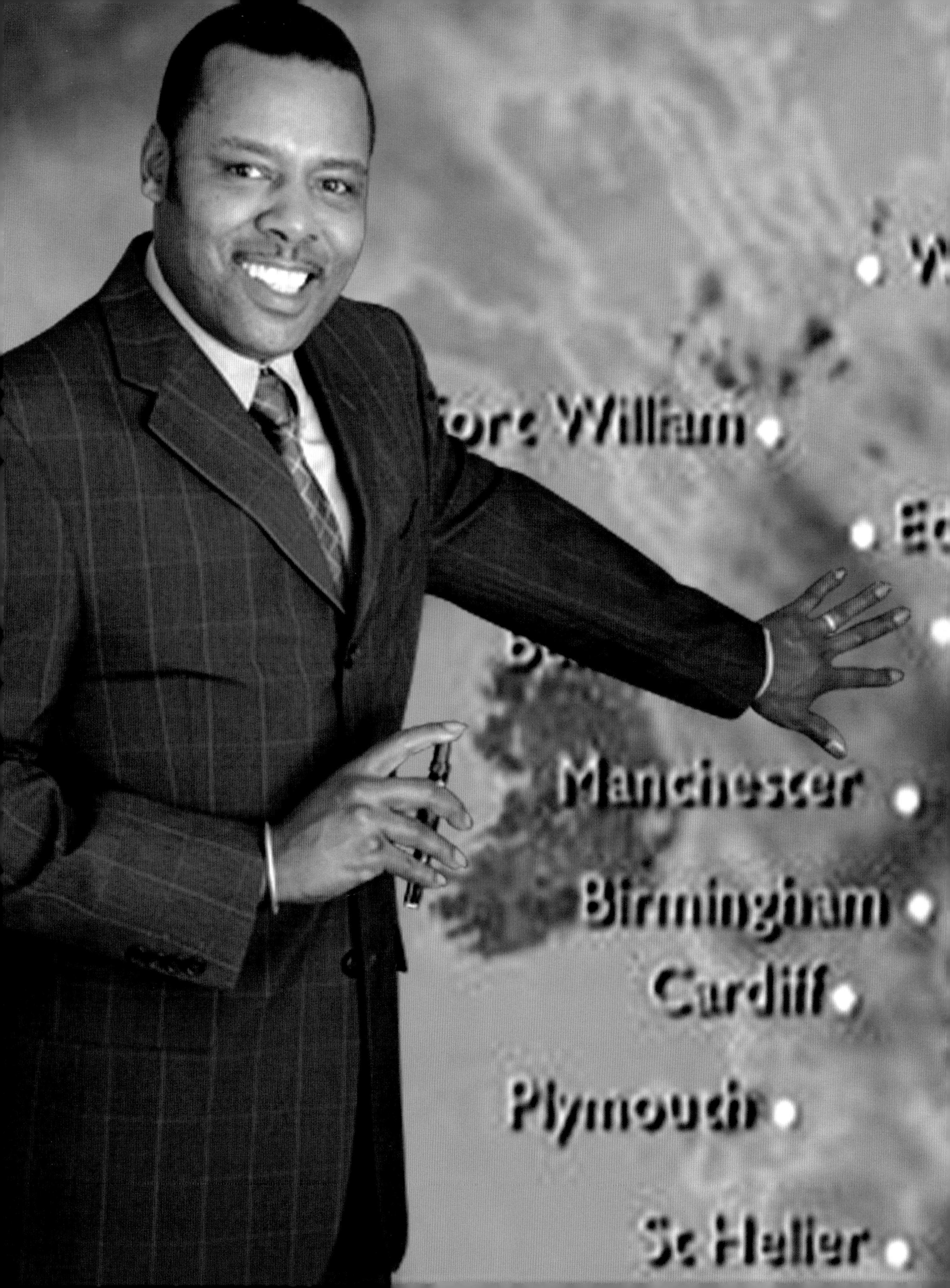

Manchester
Birmingham
Cardiff
Plymouth
St Helier

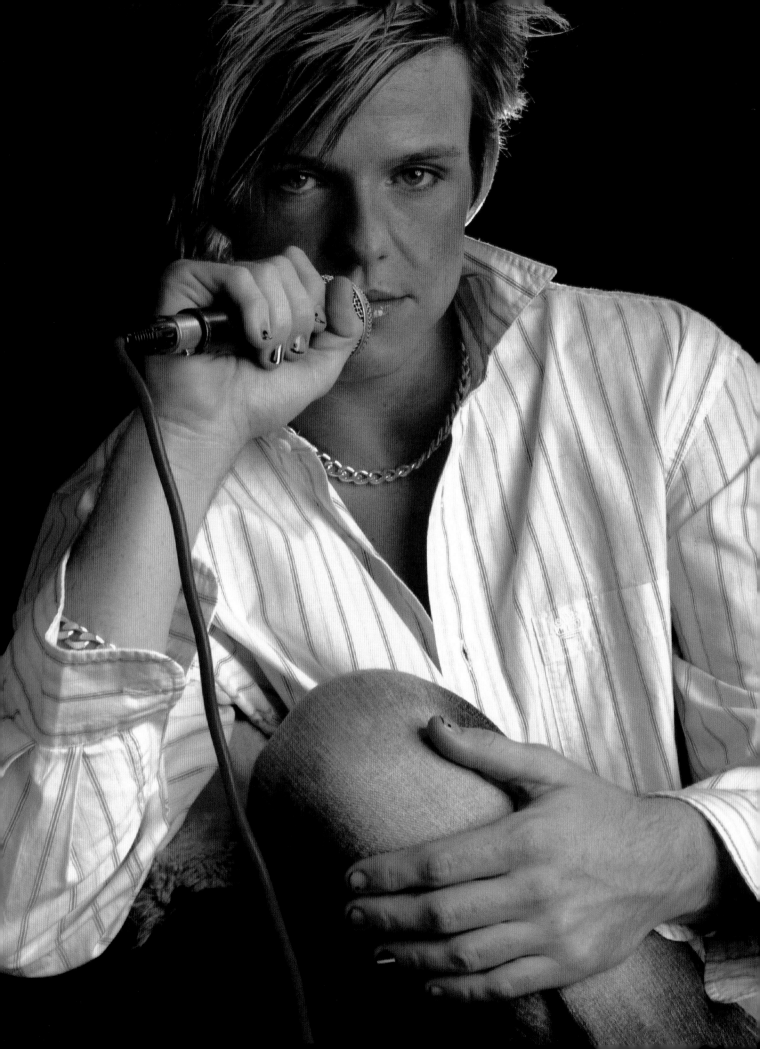

Boy band

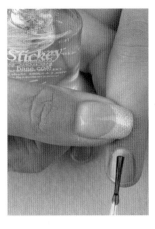

1 Even men can wear polish: many high profile celebrities have proved that over the last couple of years. Base the nails with Creative Stickey Base Coat.

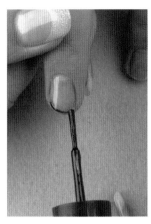

2 Take Creative Voodoo Enamel and very lightly apply a thin black line across the free edge of the nail.

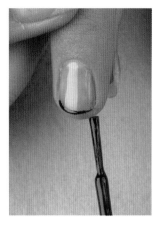

3 This can be difficult to do on short nails so clean any excess off the skin with a cotton bud and some Scrubfresh.

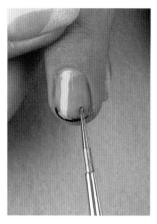

4 Using a dotting tool take a small amount of Voodoo and place a small dot at the thinner side of the black line.

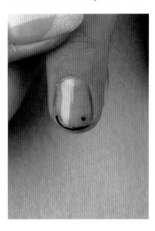

5 Once polish is dry use Super Shiney Top Coat to seal design. Do this design on nine nails.

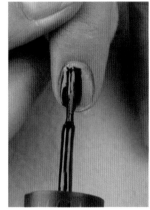

6 As a statement, make one nail different to the rest. Apply Stickey Base Coat and then two coats of Creative Voodoo Enamel.

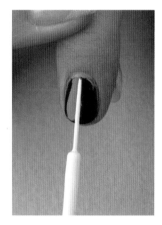

7 Take a striping brush and draw a straight line with Creative Cream Puff Enamel down the middle of the nail.

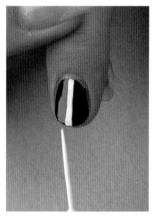

8 Neaten line if you need to with a smaller brush and allow the paint to dry.

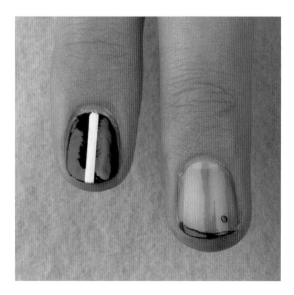

9 Apply Super Shiney Top Coat to seal. Same colours but different designs can look good together.

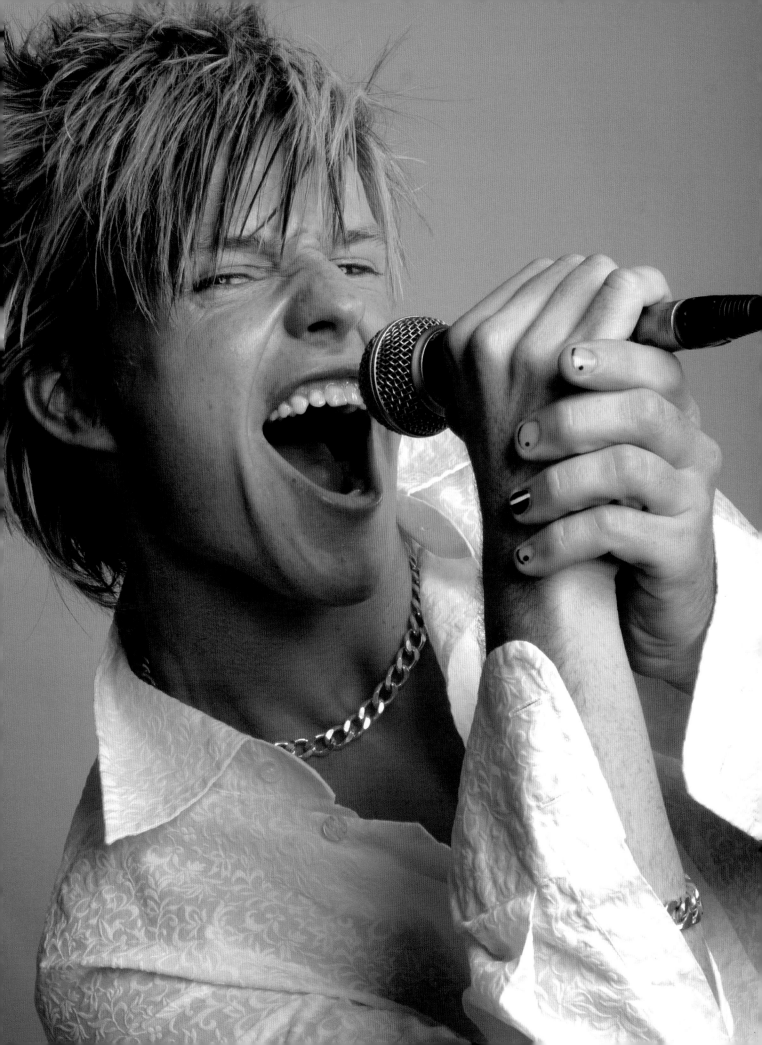

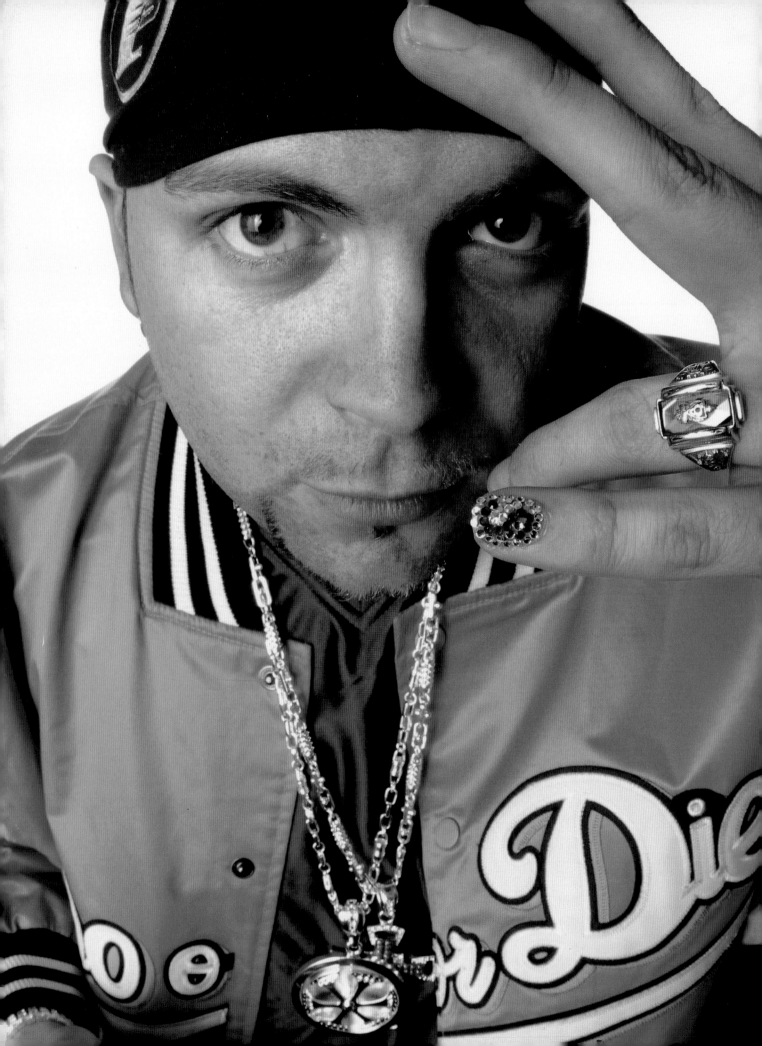

Rap artist

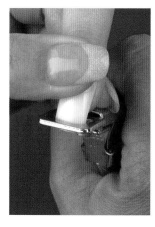

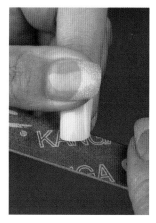

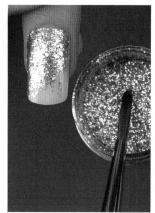

1 Dave in the main picture is actually a music artist and wanted a signature nail for the photo shoot. If your artist has not got a good length little pinky for his bling bling then add one. Apply tip with adhesive and cut to a sensible length.

2 Use a Kanga Board to shape into a square look and apply Stickey Base Coat.

3 Take a small brush and with your Stickey Base Coat and some silver glitter apply a nice even cover of glitter.

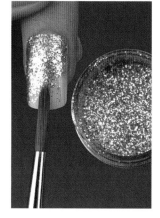

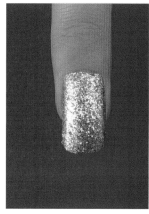

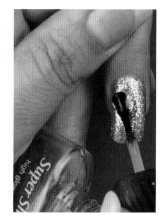

4 Start at the cuticle and work down the nail.

5 Work the glitter over the entire nail to give a good background colour.

6 Seal the glitter with Super Shiney Top Coat.

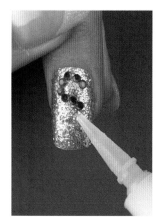

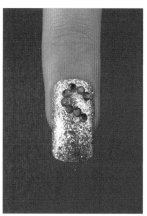

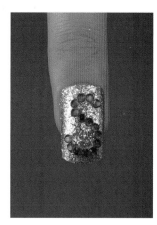

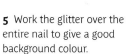

7 Apply small beads of Gel Bond in an S shape on top of the glitter.

8 Do the top half of the S first so you can see where you are going. Then with a dampened orange stick apply red rhinestones to the beads of Gel Bond.

9 Apply the second half of the rhinestones in the same way until you have a perfect S. No need to topcoat and the rhinestones should stay good on the

nail with Gel Bond. You may add rhinestones to the whole nail as in the final picture.

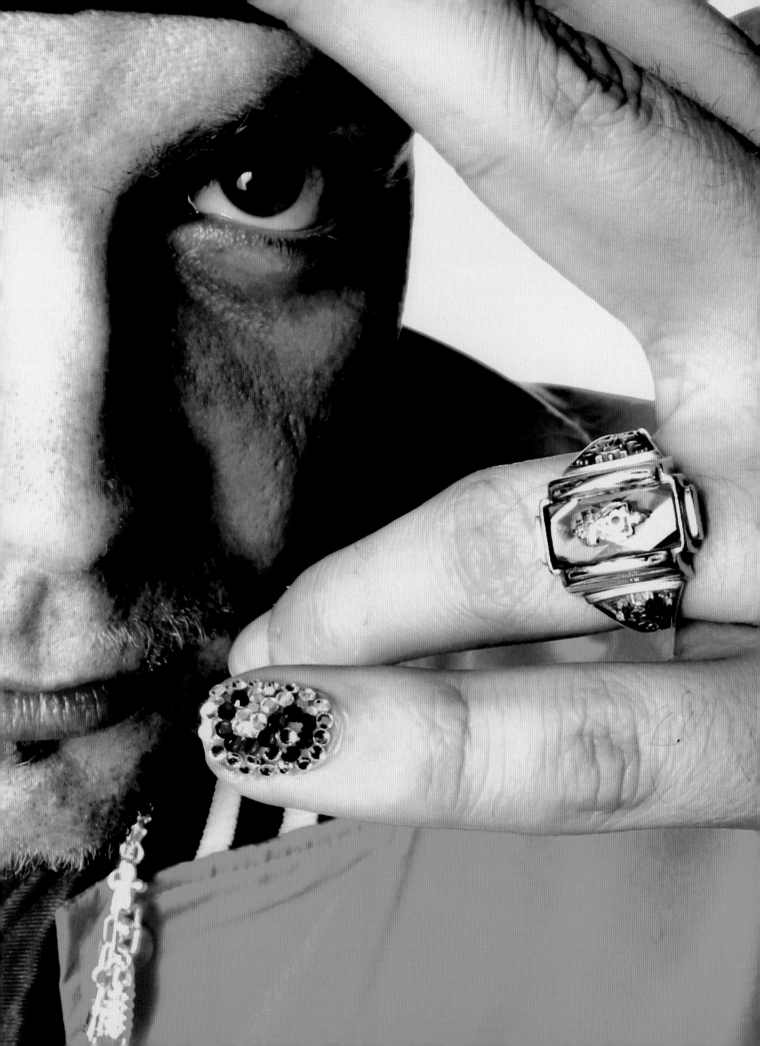

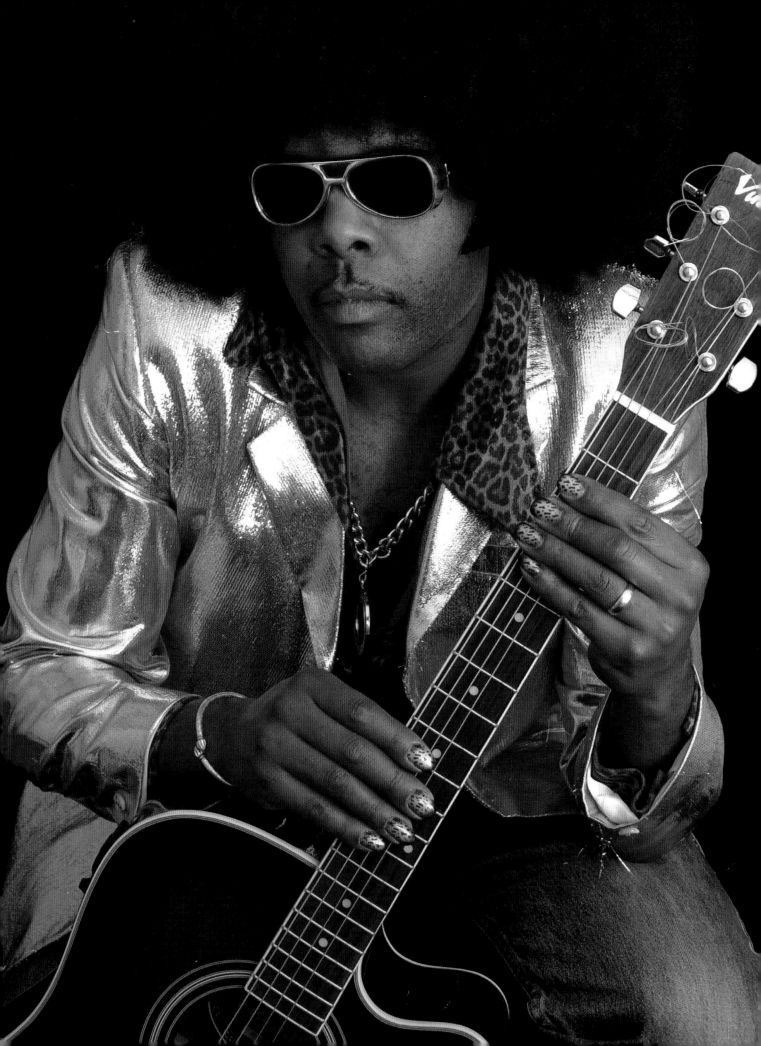

Soul man

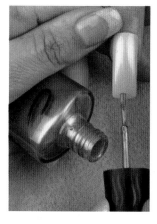

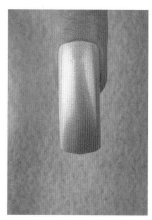

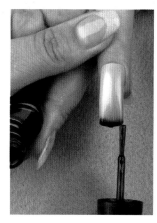

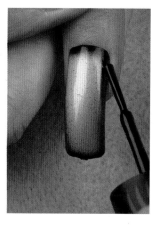

1 Apply Creative Stickey Base Coat to all nails.

2 Apply two coats of Creative Enamel to all nails.

3 Apply Creative Voodoo Enamel to the free edge of the nail.

4 Apply Voodoo around the top and sides of the nails. Do not worry too much about getting straight lines as the animal pattern will disguise this.

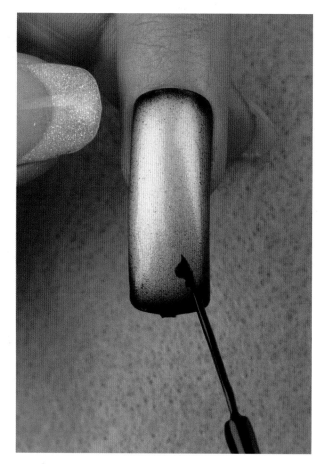

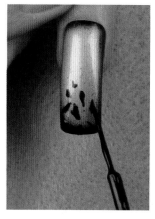

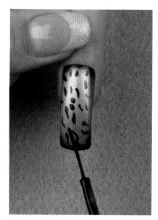

6 Work with design up the nail. Ensure that shapes are not too big. They should all be slightly different shapes.

7 Once you have completed the print go over to check there are no spaces on the nail and that all the print is even.

5 Using a small detail or striping brush use Voodoo Enamel to apply print. Start at the free edge.

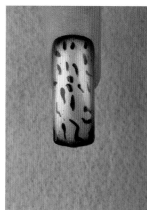

8 Once paint is dry use Creative Super Shiney Top Coat. This design can also be airbrushed very easily using a stencil.

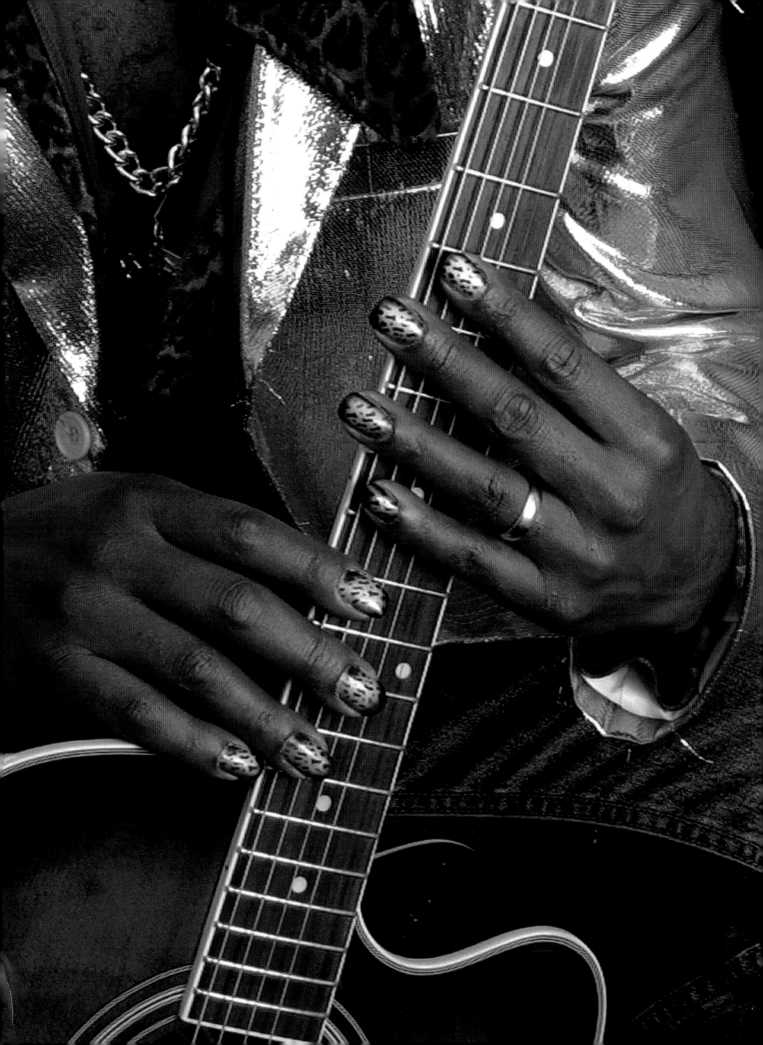

Hairdressing and beauty industry authority series – related titles

Hairdressing

Mahogany Hairdressing: Steps to Cutting, Colouring and Finishing Hair *Martin Gannon and Richard Thompson*

Mahogany Hairdressing: Advanced Looks *Richard Thompson and Martin Gannon*

Essensuals, Next Generation Toni & Guy: Step by Step

Professional Men's Hairdressing *Guy Kremer and Jacki Wadeson*

The Art of Dressing Long Hair *Guy Kremer and Jacki Wadeson*

Patrick Cameron: Dressing Long Hair *Patrick Cameron and Jacki Wadeson*

Patrick Cameron: Dressing Long Hair Book 2 *Patrick Cameron*

Bridal Hair *Pat Dixon and Jacki Wadeson*

Trevor Sorbie: Visions in Hair *Kris Sorbie and Jacki Wadeson*

The Total Look: The Style Guide for Hair and Make-up Professionals *Ian Mistlin*

Art of Hair Colouring *David Adams and Jacki Wadeson*

Begin Hairdressing: The Official Guide to Level 1 *Martin Green*

Hairdressing – The Foundations: The Official Guide to Level 2 *Leo Palladino (contribution Jane Farr)*

Professional Hairdressing: The Official Guide to Level 3 *Martin Green and Leo Palladino*

Men's Hairdressing: Traditional and Modern Barbering *Maurice Lister*

African-Caribbean Hairdressing *Sandra Gittens*

Salon Management *Martin Green*

eXtensions: The Official Guide to Hair Extensions *Theresa Bullock*

Beauty therapy

Beauty Therapy – The Foundations: The Official Guide to Level 2 *Lorraine Nordmann*

Beauty Basics – The Official Guide to Level 1 *Lorraine Nordmann*

Professional Beauty Therapy: The Official Guide to Level 3 *Lorraine Nordmann, Lorraine Williamson, Pamela Linforth and Jo Crowder*

Aromatherapy for the Beauty Therapist *Valerie Ann Worwood*

Indian Head Massage *Muriel Burnham-Airey and Adele O'Keefe*

The Official Guide to Body Massage *Adele O'Keefe*

An Holistic Guide to Anatomy and Physiology *Tina Parsons*

An Holistic Guide to Reflexology *Tina Parsons*

An Holistic Guide to Massage *Tina Parsons*

The Encyclopedia of Nails *Jacqui Jefford and Anne Swain*

Nail Artistry *Jacqui Jefford, Sue Marsh and Anne Swain*

The Complete Nail Technician *Marian Newman*

The World of Skin Care: A Scientific Companion *Dr John Gray*

Safety in the Salon *Elaine Almond*

Nutrition: A Practical Approach *Suzanne Le Quesne*

The Spa Book: The Official Guide to Spa Therapy *Jane Crebbin-Bailey, Dr John Harcup and John Harrington*